ARTHRITIS

John A. Flynn, M.D.,

Timothy Johnson, M.D.,

and

Simeon Margolis, M.D., Ph.D.

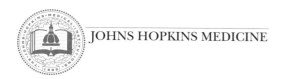JOHNS HOPKINS MEDICINE

Dear Reader:

Some 70 million Americans suffer from arthritis. There is still no cure for this painful condition, but a better understanding of its causes is aiding in the development of more effective treatments—especially new drug options that can ease the discomfort of osteoarthritis and slow the progression of rheumatoid arthritis. This White Paper reviews the most up-to-date information on the causes and treatment of arthritis and related rheumatic conditions—including drugs and surgical procedures, complementary therapies, and exercise and other self-management strategies.

Here are some of this year's highlights:

- The **best exercises** for arthritis, from a Hopkins physical therapist. (page 10)
- New finding on how to predict **progression of osteoarthritis**. (page 13)
- Why you should monitor your **blood pressure** if you take anti-inflammatory drugs. (page 15)
- Who's most likely to get **knee replacement surgery**? (page 23)
- Is **glucosamine, chondroitin, or SAM-e** effective? (page 24)
- Nine strategies for **coping with the fatigue** of arthritis. (page 33)
- **Tests you need** if you're taking medication for rheumatoid arthritis. (page 45)
- Controversy over surgery for **rheumatoid arthritis of the hand**. (page 49)

I hope that, as a result of this new understanding of how to treat arthritis, the quality of life of arthritis sufferers will be greatly enhanced in the future.

Sincerely,

John A. Flynn, M.D.
Associate Professor
Division of Rheumatology
Department of Medicine

P. S. Don't forget to visit www.HopkinsAfter50.com for the latest news on arthritis and other information that will complement your Johns Hopkins White Paper.

THE AUTHORS

John A. Flynn, M.D., M.B.A., F.A.C.P., F.A.C.R., is a graduate of the University of Missouri-Columbia School of Medicine, where the University of Missouri Medical Alumni Organization recently selected him as a recipient of the "Outstanding Young Physician Award." He completed his internship and residency in Internal Medicine at the Johns Hopkins University School of Medicine, followed by a fellowship in Clinical Rheumatology. Dr. Flynn is an Associate Professor in the Divisions of General Internal Medicine and Molecular and Clinical Rheumatology in the Department of Medicine at the Johns Hopkins University School of Medicine. He holds the D. William Schlott Professorship of Clinical Medicine and serves as the Clinical Director of the Division of General Internal Medicine. Dr. Flynn has joint appointments in the Department of Psychiatry and Behavioral Sciences as well as at the School of Nursing at Johns Hopkins University. Dr. Flynn's clinical interests include arthritis and spondyloarthropathies. His research interests include ambulatory education and the delivery of primary care in an academic setting. Dr. Flynn is a recent recipient of the "Clinician Scholar Educator Award" from the American College of Rheumatology. The award is designed to recognize and support rheumatologists dedicated to providing exemplary educational experiences for medical trainees. He has published in journals such as *Arthritis & Rheumatism, Arthritis Care & Research, The New England Journal of Medicine,* and *The Journal of General Internal Medicine.* He is co-editor of the textbook *Cutaneous Medicine.*

■ ■ ■

Simeon Margolis, M.D., Ph.D., received his M.D. and Ph.D. from the Johns Hopkins University School of Medicine and performed his internship and residency at Johns Hopkins Hospital. He is currently a professor of medicine and biological chemistry at the Johns Hopkins University School of Medicine and medical editor of *The Johns Hopkins Medical Letter: Health After 50.* He has served on various committees for the Department of Health, Education and Welfare, including the National Diabetes Advisory Board and the Arteriosclerosis Specialized Centers of Research Review Committees. In addition, he has acted as a member of the Endocrinology and Metabolism Panel of the U.S. Food and Drug Administration.

A former weekly columnist for *The Baltimore Sun,* Dr. Margolis lectures regularly to medical students, physicians, and the general public on a wide variety of topics, such as the prevention of coronary heart disease, the control of cholesterol levels, the treatment of diabetes, and the use of alternative medicine.

■ ■ ■

Timothy Johnson, M.D., an instructor in orthopedics at the Johns Hopkins University School of Medicine, contributed to the surgery sections of this White Paper.

CONTENTS

ARTHRITIS

Arthritis refers to inflammation of the joints, while rheumatic disorders include diseases of the muscles and bones as well as the joints. There are more than 100 different types of arthritis and other rheumatic disorders. This White Paper covers three common forms of arthritis—osteoarthritis, rheumatoid arthritis, and gout—as well as two other rheumatic diseases, fibromyalgia syndrome and bursitis.

Arthritis is one of the nation's most prevalent chronic health problems. An estimated one in three adults, about 70 million Americans in all, suffers from some form of arthritis. Women are particularly at risk: According to the Arthritis Foundation, arthritis affects about twice as many women as men. The annual economic cost of arthritis in the United States is estimated to be $82.5 billion. Indirect costs of arthritis, such as lost wages, account for more than three quarters of this figure.

People with arthritis can deal with their condition by learning as much as possible about its causes, effects, and treatments. A greater knowledge of arthritis makes it easier to anticipate and deal with the fluctuations in its course and find ways to overcome the physical limitations and financial problems it may cause. Physicians need to explain the rationale for treatment decisions, and patients should understand the necessity for a trial-and-error approach to treatment that uses a series of different drugs until the best one is found. Involving family members in this educational process helps them to provide support and understand any handicaps the person with arthritis might have.

ANATOMY OF THE JOINTS

A joint is where two or more bones meet, or "articulate." The ends of the bones are covered by articular cartilage, a tough but slippery material that cushions the joint and allows the bones to move smoothly. Although the word "cartilage" usually refers to articular cartilage, there is a second type of cartilage called meniscal cartilage that adds an extra layer of shock absorption to the knee in the form of two crescent-shaped pads.

The joint is sealed within a joint capsule. The outside of the joint capsule is formed by ligaments, which attach bones to other bones, and tendons, which attach muscle to bone. The synovial membrane—a thin, delicate covering on the inside of the joint capsule—secretes synovial fluid, which fills the inside of the capsule and serves as a lubricant for joint movement. Different forms of arthritis can affect each of these structures.

Osteoarthritis

Osteoarthritis (OA), also known as degenerative joint disease, is characterized by a breakdown of cartilage in the joint. This breakdown involves a roughening of cartilage, followed by pitting, ulceration, and progressive loss of cartilage surface. Unlike most of the body's tissues, which are able to regenerate, cartilage repair is hampered by a limited blood supply and the lack of an effective mechanism for cartilage regrowth.

Osteoarthritis is the most common form of arthritis. By age 40, about 90% of people have x-ray evidence of OA in the weight-bearing joints—such as the hips and knees—although symptoms generally do not begin until later in life.

While OA has little or no impact on the longevity of its sufferers (unlike some other forms of arthritis), severe involvement of the hips, knees, and spine may greatly limit activity and diminish overall quality of life for some people.

CAUSES OF OSTEOARTHRITIS

Osteoarthritis can be divided into primary or secondary OA, depending on the cause.

Primary osteoarthritis. Primary OA, the gradual breakdown of cartilage that occurs with age, is the most common type of OA. It is mostly due to stress on a joint—for example, from obesity. Obesity is especially hard on the knees: OA of the knee is nearly four times more prevalent in obese women than in normal-weight women, and nearly five times more prevalent in obese men than in normal-weight men. Genetic factors are also important. In a study of female twins, heredity contributed to 39% to 65% of hand and knee OA.

Primary OA most commonly involves the joints of the lower back, hips, knees, big toe, fingers, and base of the thumb. It can be present in just one of these joints or in all of them. The wrists, elbows, shoulders, and ankles are rarely involved.

Secondary osteoarthritis. Secondary OA, which can affect any joint, is a result of trauma, chronic joint injury due to another type

How Different Forms of Arthritis Affect the Joints

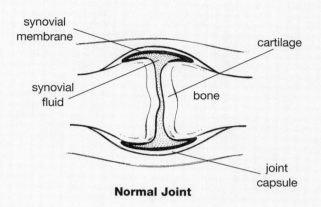

Normal Joint

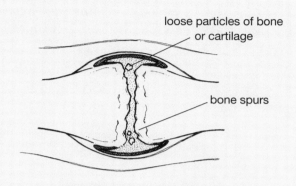

Joint With Osteoarthritis

The entire joint is enclosed in a capsule. The synovial membrane, or inner lining, of this capsule produces a slippery fluid that lubricates the space between the bones. The end of each bone is covered with resilient cartilage, which acts as a natural shock absorber. Outside the joint capsule, tendons connect bones to muscles, while the bursae produce a lubricant that eases movement between muscles and bones.

In a joint affected by osteoarthritis (the most common type of arthritis, prevalent in people over age 50), the cartilage progressively breaks down so that bone surfaces are not protected from rubbing together. The joint gradually loses its shape and alignment. The ends of the bones thicken and develop uneven bony growths, known as spurs or osteophytes. Fragments of loose cartilage or bone may float around within the joint space. All of this damage can cause pain and limit the joint's range of motion.

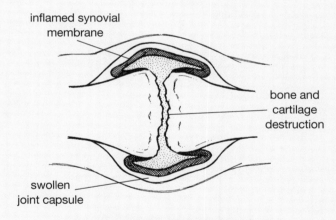

Joint With Rheumatoid Arthritis

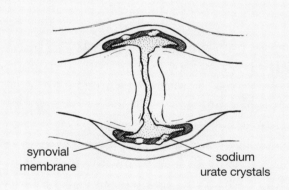

Joint With Gouty Arthritis

Rheumatoid arthritis results when—for reasons unknown—the body's immune system erroneously begins to attack tissue in the joint as if the tissue were a foreign or infectious invader. This attack results in inflammation of the synovial membrane. Inflammatory cells release enzymes that eat away at the tissues inside the joint capsule, including bone and cartilage. As with osteoarthritis, the joint loses its shape and alignment—sometimes severely so. Pain, loss of movement, and eventual destruction of the joint may ensue.

Attacks of gouty arthritis occur when excess levels of uric acid in the blood lead to the deposition of monosodium urate crystals in a joint and its synovial lining. The presence of these crystals triggers acute inflammation and pain.

of arthritis (such as rheumatoid arthritis [RA]), or overuse of the joint. The effects of joint overuse were illustrated in a 2000 study of 518 people that revealed that subjects whose jobs required at least one hour a day of kneeling or squatting were almost two times more likely to have OA in the knees than those who did not commonly perform such activities. Because trauma or overuse hastens the degeneration of cartilage, secondary OA can cause symptoms at a much younger age than primary OA.

PREVENTION OF OSTEOARTHRITIS

There are a few steps people can take to reduce their risk of both primary and secondary OA.

Primary osteoarthritis. The best way to reduce the risk of primary OA is to control one's weight. It does not take much weight loss to decrease the risk of OA. Studies have shown that overweight or obese women who lose just 11 lbs. decrease their risk of knee OA by about 50%.

In addition, several studies have shown evidence of reduced signs of OA on hip and knee x-rays in women taking estrogen replacement therapy (ERT) or hormone replacement therapy (HRT, which includes a progesterone-like hormone to lower the risk of uterine cancer from estrogen). Any protective effect disappears within 10 years of stopping the hormones, however, and does not appear to translate into reduced knee pain and disability. In any case, HRT is not recommended for this purpose, as it slightly increases the risk of heart attack, stroke, breast cancer, and blood clots in the lungs. It should be used only for the short-term relief of menopausal symptoms.

Secondary osteoarthritis. The best way to reduce the risk of secondary OA is to avoid injuring the joints. If a joint injury does occur, proper care from an orthopedic surgeon can reduce the risk of developing OA.

A number of experimental procedures are being used in an attempt to prevent OA in young people with traumatic knee injuries. The long-term success rates of these procedures are unknown. One technique involves harvesting some of the patient's own cartilage cells, having the cells cultured over several weeks, and then reimplanting them in the knee. Another involves transplanting a small graft of bone and cartilage from an area of the knee that does not bear weight to the damaged area. In addition, torn meniscal cartilage in the knee that cannot be repaired may be replaced with donor tissue, reducing the risk of damaging articular cartilage. It is important to remember that these are investigational procedures and are not used in people who already have OA or in those over 50.

SYMPTOMS OF OSTEOARTHRITIS

People rarely have symptoms of primary OA before their 40s or 50s. When symptoms first appear, they are usually mild: Morning stiffness that rarely lasts for more than 15 minutes is the only manifestation. As the disease advances, there may be mild pain when moving the affected joint. The pain is made worse by increased activity and is relieved by rest. In many people, symptoms progress no further; in others, the pain and stiffness gradually worsen until they limit daily activities, such as walking, climbing stairs, or typing. Some swelling may occur as the disease progresses, but inflammation is not a primary feature of the disease.

Enlargement of the finger joints is common in the later stages of OA. Knobby overgrowths of the joints nearest the fingertips (Heberden's nodes) occur most often in women and tend to run in families. Enlargements of the middle joints of the fingers are referred to as Bouchard's nodes.

DIAGNOSIS OF OSTEOARTHRITIS

When a patient complains of joint pain and stiffness, the doctor will obtain a complete medical history and conduct a thorough physical examination. These diagnostic procedures are important to identify the type of arthritis.

The doctor will ask questions such as:
- Which joints are involved?
- What triggers pain?
- When is pain at its worst?
- Does anything provide relief? For example, OA pain gets better with rest, whereas stiffness due to RA improves with activity.
- Have the joints been red and swollen? (This could be a sign of gout or RA.)
- Do you have morning stiffness, and how long does it last? (People with OA usually have stiffness that lasts only a few minutes in the morning; in RA, by contrast, the morning stiffness can last for hours.)

NEW RESEARCH

Torn Meniscus Increases Risk of Knee OA

Previous studies have shown that people who tear meniscal cartilage in the knee and have the entire piece of cartilage removed are at increased risk for knee osteoarthritis (OA). Now, a study finds that even people who have limited meniscectomy—removal of only the damaged cartilage— are more likely to develop OA than people without knee trauma.

Researchers assessed the symptoms and x-rayed both knees of 155 people (average age 54) who had a meniscectomy an average of 16 years earlier and of 68 age-matched controls without knee trauma. OA was present in 43% of the operated knees and 29% of the opposite knees in the meniscectomy group, and in 9% of knees in the control group. The researchers speculate that people who injure one knee may alter their gait and thus increase the risk of OA in the other knee, or that the same factors that caused the tear in one knee may also contribute to OA in the other knee.

People who had a traumatic meniscal tear were nearly three times more likely than those in the control group to have OA, and people with a degenerative tear (usually older adults) were seven times more likely. The researchers suggest that "a degenerative meniscal tear may be the first signal announcing a more widespread osteoarthritic disease in the knee joint."

ARTHRITIS AND RHEUMATISM
Volume 48, page 2178
August 2003

• What are some of your current and past work and recreational activities? (Work involving a great deal of lifting, for example, might lead to knee OA.)

The physical exam includes inspection of all the joints of the hands, arms, legs, feet, and spine to see how many are affected and whether the arthritis involves joints symmetrically (on both sides of the body). The physician may also ask questions about the person's skin, heart, lungs, eyes, and digestion, because these can be affected by some rheumatic conditions.

In most cases, the diagnosis of OA is apparent from the history and physical examination. A group of tests called an arthritis panel can be used but may give a false-positive result (indicating arthritis is present when, in fact, it is not), so it is not recommended by the American College of Rheumatology as a screening test in all people with pain or stiffness in the joints. Since no lab test can confirm the presence of OA, part of the diagnostic process involves eliminating other possibilities (called differential diagnosis).

For example, unlike RA, OA at first generally involves joints only on one side of the body and produces no signs of joint inflammation (warmth, redness, or swelling), and no generalized symptoms (fever, fatigue, and weight loss). Blood tests—such as a complete blood count (CBC), blood chemistries, and erythrocyte sedimentation rate (a measure of inflammation in the body; also known as a "sed" rate)—and urinalysis are normal. X-ray findings of a narrowed joint space and bony overgrowths called spurs help to distinguish OA from other forms of arthritis (although x-rays usually are not necessary for diagnosis). Also, marked deformity in a joint is much less common with OA than with RA or gout.

When the diagnosis is in doubt, it may be useful to obtain a sample of synovial fluid—a lubricating fluid secreted by the synovial membrane—from the affected joint. Examination of synovial fluid often can identify the type of arthritis and is essential in detecting infectious arthritis, a condition caused by a bacterial infection within the joint space. Joints with any preexisting type of arthritis are at greater risk for infection, as are the joints of people with diabetes. To obtain a sample of synovial fluid, the skin is sterilized and a local anesthetic is injected into the joint. A needle is inserted into the joint space, and a small amount of fluid is withdrawn into a syringe. The fluid is examined for the type and number of white blood cells, the presence of bacteria or other infectious agents, and the existence of uric acid crystals (suggestive of gout) to determine the cause of the joint pain.

Is Your Joint Pain Due to Osteoarthritis or Rheumatoid Arthritis?

Joint pain and stiffness are the primary symptoms of both osteoarthritis (OA) and rheumatoid arthritis (RA), and many people confuse the two. But different processes are at work in each disease. OA is a local degenerative condition resulting from the breakdown of cartilage and bone in a joint, while RA is a generalized inflammatory disease that causes swelling around the joints and can damage other organs such as the heart and lungs. The chart below outlines the main differences between OA and RA.

If you think you have OA or RA, you should contact your doctor. The doctor will ask about your medical history, perform a physical examination, and carry out tests to identify the cause of your joint pain.

	Osteoarthritis	Rheumatoid Arthritis
Age of onset	Usually begins after age 40	May begin at any age, but usually before age 50
Location of joint pain	Usually affects weight-bearing joints, such as the knees and hips, often on one side of the body only	Usually affects small joints, such as the hand, foot, wrist, elbow, shoulder, or ankle, usually on both sides of the body
Joint appearance	Usually cool, not red or swollen	Inflammation causes joints to be warm, red, and swollen
Morning joint stiffness	Lasts only a few minutes	Lasts for at least 30 minutes and can persist for hours
Symptoms besides joint pain and stiffness	Usually does not affect overall health	May be accompanied by fatigue, weight loss, and fever
Disease progression	Symptoms gradually worsen over a period of years	Symptoms worsen over a period of weeks or months
What eases pain or stiffness	Pain subsides with rest	Stiffness decreases with activity

TREATMENT OF OSTEOARTHRITIS

The rate of development and ultimate severity of OA are unpredictable. No treatment can stop or reverse its progression. But discomfort and incapacitation are not inevitable. In fact, research shows that the prognosis is generally good. One study followed 63 people with OA of the hand or knee. Based on changes in knee x-rays and reports of pain over an average of 11 years, the disease progressed little among people whose initial symptoms were mild or moderate—which is the case for most people with OA.

The goals of OA treatment are to relieve pain and maintain as much normal joint function as possible. To accomplish these goals, physicians apply a combination of treatment approaches. The most common are the careful use of medication for pain management, physical and occupational therapy to maintain flexibility and strengthen the muscles around the joint, and weight loss to decrease stress on the weight-bearing joints (consulting a nutritionist can help). In some cases, surgery may be beneficial. If possible, treatment should start with nondrug/nonsurgical options, although OA may worsen over time, eventually making surgery or long-term use of medication necessary. (By delaying the use of medications when possible, people can reduce their lifetime exposure to drugs and their side effects.)

A six-week self-help program sponsored by the Arthritis Foundation can help individuals with arthritis learn how to reduce and overcome joint pain. Studies have shown that participants in the course typically experience a 15% to 20% decline in pain, as well as significant reductions in their health care expenses over time. The effectiveness of the course may lie in its ability to improve people's understanding of the disease and to involve them in its treatment. Interested people should contact their local Arthritis Foundation chapter (see page 75); most chapters offer the program.

Weight Loss

Because excess weight puts additional stress on the joints, losing weight may be beneficial for people with osteoarthritis. In a 2000 study, researchers in North Carolina randomly assigned 21 obese people with knee OA to either an exercise program or a combination of exercise and dietary therapy. After six months, patients in the exercise group lost an average of 4 lbs. while people in the exercise and diet group lost an average of 19 lbs. Knee pain was significantly reduced in both groups, but improvements were greater among those who had lost more weight.

Heat and Ice

While drugs are effective for pain, a warm bath or shower, a heat lamp, or warm compresses also may relieve pain and ease stiffness by relaxing muscles. Paraffin (warm wax) baths can lessen pain and stiffness in the fingers and feet. In some cases, however, application of cold packs provides better relief of pain. If ice is used, it should be wrapped in a towel and applied for no longer than 20 minutes to avoid the risk of frostbite.

Using heat and cold is also a component of physical therapy. Heat can be applied to an affected joint before exercise to aid stretching and relieve minor aches. Cold packs can be applied after exercise to reduce swelling and help relieve minor pain.

Exercise

The treatment of arthritis requires both rest and exercise. The right balance between the two must be tailored to the individual and stage of the disease. While rest is important when joints ache, appropriate exercise is equally essential when symptoms subside to maintain joint motion, muscle strength, and fitness. Exercise can also help to improve balance, which may be impaired in people with knee OA.

An exercise program should be started with the approval of a physician and, preferably, under the guidance of a physical therapist who can design and teach exercises to do at home, as well as provide periodic monitoring of progress. Patience is crucial to success.

Aquatic exercise is a particularly good choice for people with arthritis because it puts little stress on the joints. Like other forms of exercise, it can increase joint flexibility, strengthen muscles, provide a good aerobic workout, and boost self-confidence.

Ideally, people should exercise nearly every day. The three forms of exercise are range of motion, muscle strengthening, and endurance (also called aerobic or "fitness" exercise).

Range-of-motion exercises. Range-of-motion exercises involve moving a joint as far as possible in every direction without causing pain. The purpose is to maintain flexibility, reduce pain and stiffness, and improve joint function. These exercises are recommended as a warm-up before a workout. For a sample of range-of-motion exercises, see the feature on pages 10–11.

Muscle-strengthening exercises. Strengthening muscles increases structural support for the joints and thereby lessens the load placed on them. Isometric exercises—pushing or pulling against a fixed object—can strengthen muscles without damaging joints, which remain immobile during the exercise. Stationary bicycling is often recommended to strengthen the muscles supporting the knees. In one study, an eight-week muscle-strengthening program improved muscle tone and decreased pain significantly in people with OA of the knee.

NEW RESEARCH

People With Arthritis Not Getting Enough Exercise

Like people without arthritis, those with arthritis are unlikely to get the recommended amount of exercise, according to a new study. Exercise is especially important for people with arthritis because it can reduce pain and disability.

To conduct the study, researchers reviewed data from a 2000 telephone survey of more than 40,000 adults. Nearly a third of the people surveyed had arthritis, and they were more likely to be physically inactive than those without arthritis (31% vs. 26%). They also found that people with arthritis were less likely to get the recommended 30 minutes of exercise on most days of the week than those without arthritis (24% vs. 27%).

The researchers were not surprised to find that people with arthritis were not getting enough exercise. Many types of exercise are painful for people with sore joints, and some people with arthritis have been inappropriately advised to avoid physical activity.

The study authors recommend that people with arthritis meet exercise recommendations by choosing "appropriate, joint-friendly types of moderate activity," such as walking, gardening, bicycling, and swimming.

ARTHRITIS AND RHEUMATISM
Volume 49, page 129
February 15, 2003

Improving Range of Motion in Arthritic Joints

Both osteoarthritis and rheumatoid arthritis can limit range of motion in the joints and lead to decreased function. A physical therapy program is a safe, effective way to maximize function by helping to maintain and even improve range of motion.

The range-of-motion exercises below are representative of those prescribed by physical therapists at Johns Hopkins Hospital. Speak to a physician or physical therapist before trying them. For the best results, perform the exercises two or three times a day. For each exercise, begin with 3 repetitions and build up to 10. Note that if the exercise calls for switching sides, one repetition includes doing the exercise on both sides.

All the exercises should be performed in a controlled, gentle manner. Your joints may feel stiff or achy during the exercises, but you should not experience any pain afterward.

—by Kelly Daley

Shoulder Sweep
- Stand with your back against a wall. Flatten your lower back against the wall by tightening your abdominal muscles.
- With your elbows straight, raise both arms out to your sides.
- Keeping your arms against the wall or as close as possible to it, raise your arms overhead in a sweeping motion. Be sure to breathe normally during the exercise.
- Return to the starting position. The entire exercise should take about four seconds.

Elbow Curl
- Stand with your arms at your sides, palms facing front.
- Keeping your elbows close to your sides, slowly raise your hands to your shoulders by bending your arms at the elbows. Then slowly lower your hands to the starting position. The entire exercise should take about four seconds.

Shoulder Rolls
- Raise your shoulders up toward your ears, then move shoulders backwards in a rolling motion. This should take approximately four seconds. You may stand or sit while doing the exercise.

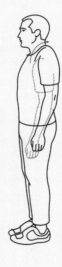

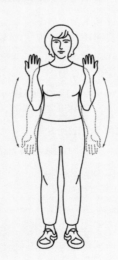

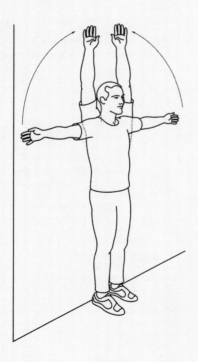

Thumb Touch
- Form an "O" with your thumb and index finger (A).
- Stretch your fingers out as wide as you can. Hold the stretch for four seconds (B).
- Touch your thumb in turn to your third, fourth, and fifth fingers, spreading your fingers wide in between each touch.
- Repeat with your other hand.

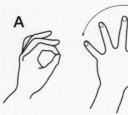

Hip Stretch

- Lie on your back on the floor or on a bed.
- Bring one knee toward your chest while keeping the other leg straight. Put your hands underneath your thigh for assistance, if necessary. Hold for a few seconds, then lower.
- Repeat with the other leg.

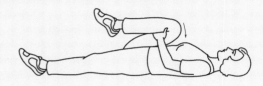

Knee Bender

- Lie on your back on the floor or on a bed with your knees bent.
- Lift one knee toward your chest. Place your hands on your shin for assistance, and gently bend the knee so that your heel approaches your buttock. Hold for a few seconds, then lower and repeat with the other leg.

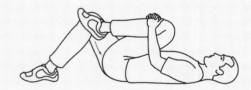

Prone Leg Lifts

- Lie face down with a pillow under your hips. Your hands should be relaxed at your sides or behind your head.
- Raise your right leg about one inch off the floor, keeping your knee straight, and hold for two seconds. Remember not to hold your breath.
- Lower and repeat with the other leg.

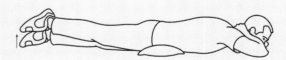

Kelly Daley is the senior physical therapist at Johns Hopkins Hospital's Department of Physical Medicine and Rehabilitation, Outpatient Physical Therapy Clinic.

Heel-to-Toe Stretch

- Sit on the edge of a chair or bed with your feet flat on the floor.
- Raise your toes as high as possible while keeping your heels on the floor.
- Hold for a few seconds, then lower your toes to the floor.
- Raise your heels up as far as possible.
- Hold for a few seconds, then lower your heels to the floor.

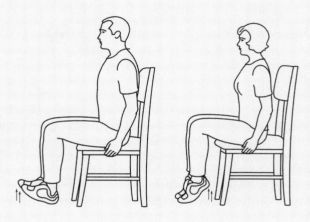

Knee Straightener

- Sit in a straight-backed chair with one foot resting on another chair or high footstool.
- Bend your knee slightly, then straighten it by pushing it down toward the floor. Hold the stretch for four seconds.
- Repeat with the other leg.

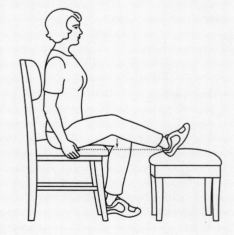

Aerobic exercises. Aerobic activities improve overall body fitness. It is possible that high-impact aerobic activities such as running might accelerate the breakdown of cartilage in weight-bearing joints (although not all studies have shown this to be the case), so most doctors recommend low- or no-impact activities such as swimming, walking, and bicycling.

People should be sure to warm up properly before exercising by walking briskly for a few minutes (to increase the heart rate) and then doing some gentle stretches (which should be easier once the muscles are warmed up). Wearing comfortable, supportive exercise shoes will help to absorb the shock of weight-bearing exercise.

Resting Joints

Resting joints involves more than simply avoiding an activity that causes pain. Equally significant are methods that reduce strain on a joint, such as using a cane, supporting the joint with a splint or brace, wearing a sling (to rest an arthritic shoulder, for example), using shoe inserts, or wearing running shoes. Although items such as canes, braces, and running shoes are available over the counter, consulting a physical or occupational therapist may prevent aggravation of arthritis symptoms caused by selecting the wrong item or using it improperly.

Drug Treatment

Pain relief usually can be achieved with acetaminophen (Tylenol). Aspirin and other nonsteroidal anti-inflammatory drugs (NSAIDs)—including ibuprofen (Advil, Motrin), naproxen (Aleve), and ketoprofen (Orudis KT), which are available over the counter—can be used if acetaminophen does not provide sufficient relief. (See the chart on pages 16–17.) In addition, a newer type of NSAID, called a cyclooxygenase-2 (COX-2) inhibitor, can be used instead of acetaminophen. COX-2 inhibitors provide pain relief similar to that of other NSAIDs but may carry a lower risk of gastrointestinal side effects. Serious side effects can still occur with COX-2 inhibitors, however, and not all studies have shown them to be safer to the stomach than traditional NSAIDs. In rare instances, corticosteroids are injected into an affected joint to relieve pain. Another option for severe pain is opiates. Trying a number of drugs may be necessary to achieve optimal pain relief.

Acetaminophen. Since inflammation plays only a minor role in OA, the anti-inflammatory effect of NSAIDs is usually not required. In most cases, OA pain can be treated with acetaminophen, which provides pain relief with fewer side effects than NSAIDs. The maximum daily dosage is 4,000 mg.

As is true with any drug, however, acetaminophen can cause dangerous side effects if taken regularly at dosages exceeding the recommended amount or if taken by people who have liver disease or drink large amounts of alcohol. Several years ago, a study linked a higher risk of end-stage kidney disease to heavy daily use of acetaminophen—no doubt leading to frustration among OA sufferers who had been told to take this drug to avoid the side effects of other pain relievers. Comparing past use of acetaminophen in 716 end-stage kidney disease patients and 361 healthy people, the study showed that taking either an average of two or more pills per day or more than 1,000 pills over a lifetime doubled the odds of end-stage kidney disease. Despite this finding, it is important to realize that acetaminophen remains the drug with the lowest overall risk of side effects. Since end-stage kidney disease is rare (only 1 of 5,000 people develop the condition each year), even regular acetaminophen users are unlikely to develop this disorder. People who use acetaminophen on a regular basis should see their doctor periodically to be monitored for side effects.

Traditional nonsteroidal anti-inflammatory drugs (NSAIDs). If nondrug measures and/or acetaminophen fail to control OA pain, NSAIDs are the next option. How well symptoms respond to a specific NSAID varies greatly from person to person. As a result, finding the right drug depends largely on trial and error, and since each drug's effects are cumulative, at least two weeks of therapy are necessary to evaluate its effectiveness. Moderate doses of NSAIDs are usually enough to control the pain of OA.

Although NSAIDs can provide effective treatment, long-term use of these drugs, even in moderate doses, can cause side effects. The most common of these effects are stomach irritation, bleeding, and ulceration caused by the drug's interference with the formation of the protective mucus that normally coats the stomach. Some degree of gastrointestinal bleeding occurs in more than half of people taking NSAIDs.

Certain groups of people—for example, those over age 65, those taking corticosteroids, and those with a history of stomach ulcers or adverse reactions to NSAIDs—are at higher risk for side effects from NSAIDs and should either be carefully monitored while taking these drugs or avoid them completely. Since NSAIDs are metabolized in the liver, people with hepatitis, cirrhosis of the liver, alcohol addiction, or other diseases that put them at greater

NEW RESEARCH

Bone Marrow Lesions May Predict Knee OA Progression

Some people with osteoarthritis (OA) of the knee have localized abnormalities in their bone marrow. These abnormalities (called bone marrow edema), along with improper alignment of the upper and lower leg bones, appear to be associated with an increased risk of knee OA progression, according to a new study.

More than 200 people with knee OA (age 45 or older) underwent magnetic resonance imaging (MRI) and x-rays at the beginning of the study, as well as 15 and 30 months later. Seventy-five participants initially showed evidence of bone marrow edema, and 36% of them had worsening OA at follow-up. Of 148 participants who did not show evidence of bone marrow edema, only 8% of them had worsening OA at follow-up. Adjusting for improper alignment of the leg bones slightly reduced the association, but OA progression was still more likely with bone marrow edema.

However, the researchers say there is no treatment for bone marrow edema and "it remains to be determined whether adding MRIs to identify bone marrow edema, long-limb radiographs to check alignment, or both to the evaluation of knee osteoarthritis adds sufficient predictive information to merit their clinical use."

ANNALS OF INTERNAL MEDICINE
Volume 139, page 330
September 2, 2003

risk for liver failure must use these drugs with care. Also, by increasing the effect of oral antidiabetes drugs, NSAIDs can lead to excessively low blood glucose (sugar) levels in people with diabetes. Because people with diabetes are also more prone to kidney disease, they should have their kidney function monitored closely while taking NSAIDs. People with asthma should be aware that NSAIDs, especially aspirin, sometimes can exacerbate the disease. And heart patients taking the anticoagulant drug warfarin (Coumadin) should not use NSAIDs because the combination may lead to excessive bleeding.

Other, less common side effects of NSAIDs are being uncovered. Large amounts of many NSAIDs (although not aspirin) may increase the risk of high blood pressure or cause kidney damage, especially in older individuals, people with heart failure or a history of kidney disease, or those taking diuretics. For example, in a nine-year study of Medicaid patients age 65 and older, those taking the largest amounts of NSAIDs had the greatest need to start therapy to lower their blood pressure. This finding does not mean that everyone using an NSAID will develop high blood pressure. Rather, the risk of the disorder is increased, and frequent NSAID users should have their blood pressure monitored regularly. In addition, people who take the osteoporosis drug alendronate (Fosamax) should use extra caution when taking NSAIDs. A small 2001 study from the *Archives of Internal Medicine* suggested that taking these drugs together may increase the risk of ulceration.

Some evidence indicates that NSAIDs may either speed the degeneration of cartilage or slow the regeneration of damaged cartilage. Another risk of NSAIDs is that by reducing pain, they may allow people to overwork their joints and cause further damage.

Avoiding NSAID side effects. All people on long-term NSAID treatment should have tests to monitor their blood count and potassium levels and to check kidney function on a regular basis. Liver function also should be tested during the first six months but usually does not need to be tested again unless the results are abnormal. People should tell their doctor if they experience any NSAID side effects, such as gastrointestinal discomfort, red blood in the stool, or black, tarry stools.

The risk of NSAID side effects can be minimized in several ways. Adequate pain relief often can be obtained with NSAIDs that have fewer side effects, such as aspirin, salsalate (Disalcid), or low-dose naproxen (Naprosyn). Tolmetin (Tolectin) and indomethacin (Indocin) should be avoided if possible because of their relatively high number of side effects. Another option is enteric-coated NSAIDs—pills specially coated to dissolve in the intestine rather than in the stomach—designed to be taken with meals.

Several medications may reduce the risk of developing an ulcer when taking NSAIDs. These agents—called cytoprotective drugs—reduce the acid content of the stomach. The disadvantages of cytoprotective drugs are that data on their effectiveness against NSAID-caused ulcers are limited, they carry side effects of their own, and they can be expensive.

The proton pump inhibitor omeprazole (Prilosec) is often used as a cytoprotective drug, but a study published in *The New England Journal of Medicine* in 2002 found a high risk (11%) of recurrent ulcer bleeding in people taking a combination of diclofenac and omeprazole.

Other cytoprotective drugs are the mucosal-coating drug sucralfate (Carafate), the histamine H_2 receptor antagonists ranitidine (Zantac), cimetidine (Tagamet), nizatidine (Axid), and famotidine (Pepcid), and the prostaglandin misoprostol (Cytotec).

Misoprostol is the only drug that has been specifically approved by the U.S. Food and Drug Administration (FDA) for use with NSAIDs to prevent stomach ulcers. Misoprostol can reduce the occurrence of ulcers in the upper part of the small intestine by two thirds and ulcers in the stomach by three fourths in regular NSAID users. Doses of misoprostol typically range from 0.1 to 0.2 mg, up to four times a day. A combination of the NSAID diclofenac and misoprostol, called Arthrotec, is also available.

COX-2 inhibitors. The COX-2 inhibitors are a newer type of NSAID that was developed to reduce the risk of stomach ulcers associated with traditional NSAIDs. The first three drugs in this class are celecoxib (Celebrex), rofecoxib (Vioxx), and valdecoxib (Bextra).

The most recent guidelines on OA from the American College of Rheumatology, published in 2000, state that some people with OA may benefit from using COX-2 inhibitors as the first-line drug treatment for moderate to severe pain. These guidelines may change as more is known about these medications and those best suited to take them. For example, a study published in *The New England Journal of Medicine* in 2002 found a high risk of recurrent ulcer bleeding in people taking celecoxib.

Traditional NSAIDs work by inhibiting two enzymes: COX-1, which is involved in the formation of prostaglandins (hormone-like substances) that help to protect against stomach ulcers, and COX-2, which produces the prostaglandins that cause inflammation. By

NEW RESEARCH

Some Arthritis Drugs Increase Risk of Cardiovascular Disease

Many anti-inflammatory drugs used to treat osteoarthritis (OA) and rheumatoid arthritis (RA) are known to increase blood pressure. This new study estimated that the small increases in blood pressure produced by these medications have a significant effect on the rates of heart attacks and strokes in people with arthritis.

The researchers used data from the Framingham study on the relationship between blood pressure and cardiovascular events (like heart attacks and strokes) and data indicating that 11.8 million adults with OA or RA in the United States receive medication to treat high blood pressure. The researchers then estimated that a 1-mm Hg increase in systolic blood pressure (the top number in a blood pressure reading) in these people would cause 7,100 more cardiovascular events each year. A 5-mm Hg increase in their systolic blood pressure would cause 35,700 additional cardiovascular events yearly.

According to an accompanying editorial, doctors should vigilantly monitor blood pressure in their arthritis patients and try to prescribe arthritis medications that are less likely to increase blood pressure.

THE JOURNAL OF RHEUMATOLOGY
Volume 30, pages 642 and 714
April 2003

Commonly Used Nonsteroidal Anti-Inflammatory Drugs (NSAIDs) 2004

Drug Type	Generic Name	Brand Name	Average Daily Dosage*
Acetylsalicylic acid	aspirin	Anacin Bayer Bufferin Easprin ZORprin	3,600 to 5,400 mg
Nonacetylated salicylates	choline magnesium trisalicylate salsalate	Trilisate Disalcid	3,000 mg 1,000 to 3,000 mg
COX-2 inhibitors	celecoxib rofecoxib valdecoxib	Celebrex Vioxx Bextra	OA: 200 mg RA: 200 to 400 mg OA: 12.5 to 25 mg RA: 25 mg 10 mg
Enolic acid	meloxicam	Mobic	7.5 to 15 mg
Fenamate	meclofenamate sodium	—	200 to 400 mg
Acetic acid	diclofenac sodium diclofenac/misoprostol etodolac indomethacin sulindac tolmetin sodium	Voltaren Arthrotec Lodine Indocin Clinoril Tolectin	100 to 150 mg OA: 150 mg/0.6 mg RA: 225–300 mg/0.6–0.8 mg 800 to 1,200 mg 50 to 200 mg 300 to 400 mg 1,200 to 1,800 mg
Naphthylalkanone	nabumetone	Relafen	1,000 to 2,000 mg
Propionic acid derivatives	fenoprofen calcium ibuprofen ketoprofen naproxen naproxen sodium	Nalfon Advil Motrin Orudis Naprosyn Anaprox	900 to 3,200 mg 800 to 2,400 mg 200 to 300 mg 440 to 1,500 mg 440 to 1,500 mg

* These dosages represent an average range for the treatment of arthritis. The precise effective dosage varies from patient to patient and depends on many factors. Do not make any changes in your medication without consulting your doctor.

† Average wholesale prices to pharmacists for 100 tablets or capsules (unless otherwise indicated) of the dosage strength listed. Costs to consumers are higher. If a generic version is available, the cost is listed in parentheses. Source: *Red Book, 2003* (Medical Economics Data, publishers).

‡ Cost of the over-the-counter version.

Wholesale Cost (Generic Cost)†	Comments
400 mg: $8‡ (325 mg: $2) 325 mg: $6‡ (325 mg: $2) 325 mg: $3‡ (325 mg: $2) 975 mg: $59 (325 mg: $2) 800 mg: $98 (325 mg: $2)	Least expensive NSAID. Enteric-coated formulation lessens gastrointestinal problems because it dissolves in the intestine rather than the stomach. Alters blood-clotting function, which may lead to bleeding.
500 mg: $104 (500 mg: $62) 750 mg: $135 (750 mg: $38)	These drugs tend not to damage the stomach lining and may be especially useful for elderly people at risk for gastrointestinal bleeding or ulcers. May also be good for people with impaired kidney function or those who must also take diuretics. May be less effective pain relievers than other NSAIDs.
100 mg: $158 200 mg: $276 12.5 mg: $276 25 mg: $276 10 mg: $293 20 mg: $293	These drugs were formulated to reduce the risk of ulcers and other gastrointestinal side effects, and the FDA allows the manufacturers of rofecoxib to make this claim in comparison with naproxen, but not all studies have shown them to be safer on the stomach than traditional NSAIDs. They have also been associated with heart problems, kidney damage, aseptic meningitis, and slow healing of bone fractures in animals.
7.5 mg: $257 15 mg: $299	Used specifically for the pain and stiffness of osteoarthritis. Serious side effects, such as gastrointestinal bleeding, are rare.
(100 mg: $340)	May cause bowel irritation that could progress to more serious colitis in a small percentage of people.
50 mg: $143 (50 mg: $92) 50 mg/0.2 mg: $184 400 mg: $180 (400 mg: $148) 50 mg: $110 (50 mg: $55) 150 mg: $123 (150 mg: $97) 400 mg: $159 (400 mg: $110)	These drugs (especially indomethacin) can cause central nervous system side effects, such as forgetfulness or convulsions. However, indomethacin can be very effective for severe arthritis of the hip in people who are not good candidates for surgery. Diclofenac/misoprostol is sometimes used by people at high risk for developing NSAID-induced ulcers.
500 mg: $147 (500 mg: $133) 750 mg: $173 (750 mg: $153)	Studies suggest that nabumetone does not cause stomach ulceration or damage to the gastrointestinal tract in the elderly and appears to pose little or no threat to the kidneys.
300 mg: $54 (600 mg: $57) 200 mg: $10‡ (200 mg: $4) 200 mg: $5‡ (200 mg: $4) 50 mg: $123 (50 mg: $104) 250 mg: $106 (250 mg: $80) 275 mg: $101 (275 mg: $85)	Fenoprofen is the only NSAID that should not be taken with food. Ibuprofen is available in generic form by prescription as well as over the counter (Advil and Motrin). Ketoprofen is available over the counter as Orudis KT, and naproxen is available over the counter as Aleve.

inhibiting COX-2 and sparing COX-1, these new drugs are theorized to treat pain and inflammation like older NSAIDs but with fewer adverse gastrointestinal effects. In fact, the FDA allows the manufacturers of rofecoxib to promote this medication as being safer for the stomach than naproxen. Not all studies have shown COX-2 inhibitors to be safer for the stomach than other NSAIDs, however. Part of the problem is that many of the studies in support of the COX-2 inhibitors have been sponsored by their manufacturers and may be biased. Additional studies and independent analyses will be required to determine exactly what the benefits and risks may be.

There are several risks associated with COX-2 inhibitors. Rofecoxib has been linked to serious cardiovascular problems, such as heart attacks, angina, and high blood pressure. (Note: Some doctors prescribe low-dose aspirin to guard against the increased rate of cardiovascular problems, but this may negate any reduced risk of gastrointestinal complications.) It has also been associated with kidney failure and aseptic meningitis, an inflammation of the membranes covering the brain and spinal cord. Finally, studies in animals have shown that COX-2 inhibitors may seriously impair the ability of bone fractures to heal.

Hyaluronan. Viscosupplementation is a relatively new treatment option for people with OA of the knee. The procedure involves the injection of hyaluronan, a natural component of synovial fluid, directly into the knee joint. It may provide pain relief and improvements in knee function for up to one year, but its long-term effects are unknown.

The FDA has currently approved three hyaluronan derivatives for the treatment of knee OA. Hyalgan and Supartz, two brands of sodium hyaluronate, are injected into the knee once a week for five weeks. Synvisc, the brand name for hylan G-F 20, is administered three times, with one week between each injection. The cost for a complete series of injections is about $500. If the results of initial therapy are unsatisfactory, a second course of injections about eight months later may prove more beneficial.

One major advantage of viscosupplementation is that it appears to have few, if any, serious side effects. The most common side effects are local reactions at the injection site, such as pain, swelling, rash, and itching; these reactions are temporary and may result from the injections rather than the agent itself.

For now, viscosupplementation has a limited role in the treatment of OA. It should be considered only by people who cannot tolerate basic pain relievers like acetaminophen or anti-inflammatory medications, who are unable to have joint replacement surgery, or who wish to delay surgery if possible.

Corticosteroid injection. People who cannot take NSAIDs or acetaminophen, or who have taken them and have not benefited, may wish to have a corticosteroid injection into the joint. This treatment provides pain relief but does not reverse the underlying degenerative process in the joint.

Injection of corticosteroids directly into the joint may also help someone who experiences an acute worsening of OA symptoms or is a poor candidate for joint replacement surgery. This technique can also provide temporary relief from discomfort and increased mobility for special situations, such as a parent wanting to dance at a child's wedding. Corticosteroids relieve pain by reducing inflammation, and one injection can provide pain relief for a few weeks to several months—enough time to initiate physical therapy. Pain returning within a few weeks may indicate a problem other than inflammation.

Because frequent corticosteroid injections increase the risk of damage to the cartilage, they should be performed no more than two or three times a year.

Other injections. Eventually, other types of injections may become available. One small study found that injections of 1 mg of morphine into the knee joint of people with OA provided pain relief for at least one week. Additional studies might find that injection of longer-acting pain medication results in more prolonged relief.

Tidal irrigation. Tidal irrigation is sometimes used to treat OA of the knee. In this procedure, a saline solution is repeatedly injected into and then withdrawn from the joint space. The goal is to break up areas where the synovial membrane has attached to itself, and it may also help to remove debris from the joint. The American College of Rheumatology currently does not recommend tidal irrigation, citing the need for further study.

Surgery

A number of surgical procedures may be helpful when arthritis is severely disabling. These include joint replacement, arthroscopy, arthrodesis, osteotomy, and hemicallotasis.

Joint replacement (arthroplasty). The most common type of arthroplasty is total joint replacement, in which the entire diseased or damaged joint is removed and replaced with a mechanical one (a prosthesis) to relieve pain and restore function. Between 80% and 90% of joint replacements are of the hip and knee, although

NEW RESEARCH

Glucosamine/Chondroitin Safe for People With Arthritis and Diabetes

While animal studies have shown that supplements containing glucosamine can raise blood glucose levels, a new study is the first to suggest that these supplements are safe for people with both osteoarthritis (OA) and diabetes.

The study included 34 people (average age 70) with OA and type 2 diabetes who were taking one or two diabetes medications. Twenty-two participants took a glucosamine/chondroitin combination containing 1,500 mg of glucosamine and 1,200 mg of chondroitin sulfate; the other 12 participants took a placebo.

Three months later, neither group had a significant change in hemoglobin A1c levels (a measure of blood glucose control over the previous two to three months). One person in the supplement group discontinued treatment because of excessive flatulence.

The study did not address whether the treatment is beneficial for people with OA, but the authors conclude that "since patients with diabetes are at risk for toxic effects from some of the current treatments for osteoarthritis (NSAIDs in particular), glucosamine may provide a safe alternative treatment for these patients."

ARCHIVES OF INTERNAL MEDICINE
Volume 163, page 1587
July 14, 2003

joints in the shoulder, elbow, hand, ankle, and foot also can be replaced. New technology and improved operative techniques and materials have made joint replacement the best treatment for many people. Each year approximately 150,000 joints are replaced in the United States, primarily (but not exclusively) for arthritis sufferers. For hip replacement—the most common type—the success rate is almost 95% during the first 5 to 10 years, according to the Arthritis Foundation.

Most artificial joints are made out of cobalt chrome or a titanium alloy and lined with a medical-grade plastic called ultra-high-molecular-weight polyethylene. The polyethylene lining keeps the joints moving smoothly but tends to wear away with time. In 2002, the FDA approved two new hip implants that are lined with a durable ceramic instead of plastic in an attempt to reduce this deterioration.

Before considering surgery, people should consult their physician about more conservative treatments—including rest, ice or heat, muscle-strengthening exercises, and pain medication.

Reasons for joint replacement include the following:
• Failure of arthritis to respond adequately to the various anti-arthritic drugs or drug combinations and lifestyle changes within six months;
• Joint pain severe enough to cause awakening at night;
• Joint pain that limits walking to about one block; and
• Evidence of substantial joint degeneration on x-ray, but only if accompanied by severe pain. (Even when x-rays show significant joint deterioration, some people with arthritis have little or no pain.)

If arthroplasty is deemed necessary, patients should get as much information as they can about the procedure, recovery, and rehabilitation. In one study, people who participated in a two-hour educational program prior to knee replacement showed markedly greater and faster improvement after surgery than another group of people who had the same operation but did not participate in the program. The people in the educational program spent an average of two fewer days in the hospital and required fewer sessions of physical therapy to attain full recovery.

To ensure the most satisfaction from the results of arthroplasty, patients should discuss with their surgeon before the operation the kinds of activities (including sports) they intend to continue afterward. This information will aid the surgeon in selecting the type of prosthesis, implantation technique, and rehabilitation, as well as making the patient more aware of the risks and limitations of his or

Relief With Topical Analgesics

If you have mild to moderate osteoarthritis, over-the-counter creams and ointments may help ease the pain.

Topical analgesics are nonprescription products that are applied to the skin over an aching joint to provide temporary relief of pain. They can be useful for people with mild to moderate osteoarthritis pain who experience inadequate pain relief with acetaminophen (Tylenol) or wish to avoid the side effects of oral pain relievers.

The three main types of topical analgesics are counterirritants, salicylates, and capsaicin; combination products are also available. They are usually sold as creams, gels, or ointments that are gently rubbed into the skin, but sprays and patches are also available.

Topical nonsteroidal anti-inflammatory drugs such as ketoprofen, felbinac, ibuprofen, and piroxicam are popular in Europe and the United Kingdom but have yet to become commercially available in the United States.

Counterirritants
Counterirritants contain such ingredients as menthol, camphor, eucalyptus oil, and turpentine oil. When applied to the skin over an affected joint, they mask pain by producing a warm or cool sensation. These preparations can be applied to the skin three or four times a day. A frequent side effect is reddening of the skin, which is harmless and temporary.

Salicylates
Oral salicylates (aspirin) and topical salicylates, such as trolamine salicylate or methyl salicylate, reduce pain and inflammation by inhibiting the release of prostaglandins. An analysis in the *British Medical Journal* concluded that topical preparations relieve pain more effectively than a placebo, but it is unknown how they compare with oral pain medications.

Salicylates can be applied to the skin up to four times a day. Because some of the medication is absorbed into the body, people who are sensitive to aspirin or other salicylates or are taking medication that might interact with them—for example, warfarin (Coumadin)—should use these creams with caution. Symptoms of salicylate toxicity, including ringing in the ears, blurred vision, and shortness of breath, should be reported to a doctor.

Capsaicin
Other topical preparations contain capsaicin, the compound that gives hot peppers their "bite." This compound reduces the amount of a neurotransmitter called substance P, which is thought to release inflammation-causing enzymes and possibly trigger pain impulses to the brain. The ointment should be applied to affected joints three or four times a day. It usually takes one to two weeks for pain to diminish, although up to six weeks of treatment might be required for maximum benefit. Pain quickly returns after capsaicin is discontinued. Burning, stinging, and redness occur in 40% to 70% of people, but these side effects usually diminish after several days of use.

General Precautions
Topical treatments for joint pain are not dangerous and have few side effects, but some precautions apply. The medications are for external use only and should not come in contact with the eyes, nose, mouth, or any open skin. The products should be used no more than three or four times a day and should be discontinued immediately if severe irritation develops. If symptoms do not improve after seven days, most manufacturers recommend discontinuing the product and seeing a doctor. In addition, many of the products come with warnings not to bandage or apply heat to a treated area.

Some topical preparations also contain glucosamine or chondroitin, but there is no evidence that these compounds have any effect on osteoarthritis when applied to the skin. A recent randomized controlled study of 63 people found that one such preparation was more effective than placebo in relieving the pain of knee OA within four weeks, but this effect was most likely explained by the product's active ingredient: camphor. This study was published in March 2003 in *The Journal of Rheumatology*.

Common Brands
The following are some common brands of topical analgesics. All are available over the counter.

Counterirritants:
Flexall 454 Maximum Strength Gel
Therapeutic Mineral Ice
Combination products:
ArthriCare
BenGay
Flexall 454 Ultra Plus Gel
Icy Hot Chill Stick

Salicylates:
Aspercreme
Sportscreme
Capsaicin:
Capzasin-HP
Capzasin-P
Zostrix
Zostrix-HP

her chosen activities. Recommended activities after surgery include golfing, swimming, cycling, bowling, and sailing. Not recommended are such activities as running, racquetball, and basketball.

Arthroplasty requires hospitalization and, usually, general anesthesia. (In some cases, spinal anesthesia to numb the lower body may be used for knee replacement.)

Joint replacement options. Two types of hip and knee joint replacements are available: cemented and uncemented. Cemented joints are glued to the natural bone; uncemented joints are covered with a porous, "bumpy" material into which the natural bone eventually grows and attaches itself. About 90% of artificial joints last 10 to 15 years, after which a second joint replacement (called a revision) can be implanted.

Cemented joints are the best choice for people with weaker bones because the cement holds the device firmly in place. They are more difficult to revise than uncemented joints because the cement needs to be removed. They are usually used in older, frailer patients, who not only are more likely to have thinner bones but are less likely to need a revision.

Uncemented joints are usually the best choice for younger, healthier patients, who are more likely to need a revision and who usually have the dense bone needed to keep the device firmly in place. As many as 30% of people with uncemented total hip prostheses develop thigh pain, but this usually goes away in two to three years.

Revisions tend to be riskier and technically more difficult operations than the initial replacement surgery. The revision procedure is basically a more complicated version of the first one: More bone is cut away, the surgery takes longer, and blood loss is greater. In addition, since revisions take place up to 20 years after the original surgery, patients are older and perhaps less healthy.

Significant complications occur in about 5% of joint replacements. The most frequent is blood clots in leg veins, although surgeons take extra precautions to help prevent this problem by using aspirin, heparin, or similar blood thinners or leg compression devices (typically a pneumatic compression device that repeatedly inflates and deflates to massage the leg). A potentially more serious but less common complication is infection, which usually requires removal of the prosthesis and several weeks in the hospital for antibiotic therapy. Eventually, a new prosthesis is implanted. Arthroplasty patients must guard against infection for as long as one to two years after surgery by taking oral antibiotics for even small infections and before dental work or urinary examinations. With preventive measures, the infection rate is no more than 3%.

Rehabilitation. Pain may be considerable immediately after the surgery—from muscles disturbed during the operation, rather than from the joint itself. Rehabilitation begins in the hospital, usually the day after surgery. Recovery from a hip replacement is 80% complete within four weeks and 100% complete within six months. Recovery from a knee replacement is 80% complete within four weeks and 100% complete after one year. During this time, a strict timetable of exercise, rest, and medication is crucial to the success of the surgery.

Continuous passive motion may be used when the knee joint is replaced. This therapy utilizes a device that slowly but continuously bends and straightens the patient's leg for several hours a day, gradually increasing the range of movement. Watching television or talking with visitors is possible while using the device. Some people are able to read during therapy, although others find the machine to be too distracting.

Recovery from all types of joint replacement requires a series of sessions with a physical therapist. Physical therapy focuses on building back strength and regaining flexibility. The physical therapist may use techniques such as massage and application of cold to minimize swelling, which interferes with flexibility. Patients are given a series of exercises to perform at home.

Research shows that the success of arthroplasty depends greatly on the motivation and participation of the patient after the operation. In fact, the decision to have joint replacement surgery should be accompanied by a commitment to a period of recuperation. Successful joint replacement, especially knee replacement, requires a considerable investment of time and energy in postsurgical rehabilitation, but the rewards are great. Studies of joint replacement patients have shown improvements in psychological well-being and life satisfaction, as well as reduced pain.

Resurfacing. Resurfacing, also referred to as bone relining, is a type of joint replacement. In this procedure, the damaged cartilage and bone ends in the hip joint are removed and capped with metal; the joint capsule is sometimes lined with plastic. This procedure is not widely used.

Unicompartmental knee replacement. Unlike total knee replacement, unicompartmental knee replacement is a procedure in which only the damaged section of the knee is replaced. It may be an option for people with limited knee damage, but it is rarely used

NEW RESEARCH

Knee Arthroplasty Rates Differ by Race, Gender, Geography

Whites are more likely to have knee arthroplasty than blacks or Hispanics, and the disparity is greater in some parts of the United States than in others, according to a new study.

Researchers reviewed data on more than 400,000 knee arthroplasties performed on Medicare recipients between 1998 and 2000. Overall, the annual national rate for the procedure was higher for white women (6 procedures per 1,000 women) than for Hispanic women (5.4 procedures) and black women (4.8 procedures). The annual rates were also higher for white men (4.8 procedures per 1,000 men) than for Hispanic men (3.5 procedures) and black men (1.8 procedures). The higher rate of knee arthroplasty in women was expected because women are diagnosed with osteoarthritis more often than men.

Geography also played a role. For example, the knee arthroplasty rate in Philadelphia was almost twice as high for white men as for black men, but it was more than three times higher for white men than black men in Memphis.

The researchers speculate that patient preferences may affect the rate of knee arthroplasty. They say that educating people with osteoarthritis about the potential benefits of surgery may help address the disparity in care.

THE NEW ENGLAND
JOURNAL OF MEDICINE
Volume 349, pages 1350 and 1379
October 2, 2003

Supplements for Osteoarthritis

Many people take glucosamine, chondroitin, or SAM-e for their osteoarthritis. Do any of these remedies really work?

Americans spend more money each year on natural remedies for osteoarthritis (OA) than for any other medical problem. Alternative therapies can be appealing, especially when conventional medications such as acetaminophen (Tylenol) and nonsteroidal anti-inflammatory drugs (NSAIDs) don't sufficiently relieve symptoms. Two of the most popular supplements for OA are glucosamine and chondroitin. Some people with OA take S-adenosylmethionine (SAM-e) in an effort to relieve symptoms. But are these supplements safe and effective treatments for OA?

Glucosamine and Chondroitin

OA is characterized by a gradual deterioration of cartilage in the joints. The breakdown is due in part to the loss of proteoglycans, components of cartilage that help absorb the shock of body movements and provide the joints with strength and elasticity. The release of cartilage-degrading enzymes by cells in the joint known as chondrocytes also contributes to the deterioration.

Glucosamine and chondroitin occur naturally in the body, and both play an important role in the formation and maintenance of cartilage. When glucosamine and chondroitin are taken as supplements, it's not known how they work to treat OA, but it is thought that they might stimulate the formation of new proteoglycans and inhibit the production of cartilage-degrading enzymes. These effects, in turn, may stimulate the production of new cartilage and help the body repair damaged cartilage. The two compounds may also have anti-inflammatory properties.

A January 2003 review article in *American Family Physician* suggested that glucosamine and chondroitin reduce the symptoms of OA, but there is no evidence that the supplements slow disease progression or regenerate damaged cartilage. The review also concluded that glucosamine and chondroitin cause fewer gastrointestinal side effects than NSAIDs. People often take glucosamine and chondroitin together, but the combination appears to be no better than taking either supplement separately.

The National Institutes of Health is currently conducting a clinical trial comparing glucosamine, chondroitin, a glucosamine/chondroitin combination, celecoxib (Celebrex), and a placebo in the treatment of knee OA pain. Results are expected in 2005. In the meantime, the American College of Rheumatology does not recommend the use of supplements for OA. If you do decide to take glucosamine or chondroitin, do not stop taking proven treatments such as

because most results have been poor.

Arthroscopy. Arthroscopy entails the insertion of an arthroscope—a thin, lighted tube with a camera attached to one end—into a joint. This procedure is performed by an orthopedic surgeon in a hospital operating room or an outpatient surgical suite. It may be used diagnostically (to determine the type of arthritis or the amount of damage) or therapeutically (to perform debridement or lavage). Debridement involves smoothing roughened cartilage, while lavage involves flushing out the joint to remove debris. A recent study found that neither debridement nor lavage are effective treatments for knee OA, but arthroscopy may still be useful for some people with large pieces of debris or torn cartilage. Arthroscopy can be used on the knee, hip, shoulder, elbow, or hand.

Arthrodesis. In this procedure, a surgeon fuses together two bones in a finger, wrist, ankle, or foot joint. While this operation results in a loss of flexibility, it relieves the pain caused by two bones rubbing against each other in a damaged joint. The fused bone is more stable and can bear weight much better than before. This acetaminophen or NSAIDs.

Glucosamine is made from the shells of crustaceans, so people who are allergic to shellfish should not take this supplement. To prevent excessive bleeding, chondroitin should not be taken together with the anti-coagulant drug warfarin (Coumadin). In addition, people with diabetes should be especially cautious when using glucosamine. Although a small recent study suggests that these supplements may be safe for people with diabetes (see the sidebar on page 19), it is still possible that the supplements may elevate blood glucose levels. Check with your doctor.

Glucosamine and chondroitin should be taken in pill form; topical products containing chondroitin and glucosamine are not likely to relieve arthritis pain, since these substances are too large to be absorbed through the skin. The suggested daily doses are 1,500 mg of glucosamine or 1,200 mg of chondroitin.

Supplements are not regulated by the U.S. Food and Drug Administration (FDA), so there is no guarantee that any product contains the amount of active ingredient indicated on the label. However, a recent study of glucosamine and chondroitin found that 15 products contained at least 90% of the amount of the active ingredient listed on the label. The three least expensive combination products that were accurately labeled were: Puritan's Pride Maximum Strength Glucosamine Chondroitin; Spring Valley Glucosamine Chondroitin Double Strength; and The Vitamin Shoppe Glucosamine and Chondroitin Sulfate. The least expensive, accurately labeled individual supplements were Spring Valley Glucosamine Complex (for glucosamine only) and Twinlab CSA (for chondroitin only). The greatest benefit results from using the suggested daily doses mentioned above rather than the ones suggested by the manufacturers.

SAM-e

SAM-e, a substance naturally present in the body, is involved in many biochemical reactions, including the synthesis of cartilage. Used for decades in Europe as a treatment for depression and arthritis, SAM-e was introduced as an over-the-counter supplement in the United States in 1999. Because the quality of the studies of SAM-e for OA is questionable, SAM-e is not recommended as a treatment for OA.

General Precautions

Glucosamine, chondroitin, and SAM-e are all available without a prescription in pharmacies and health food stores, but this does not mean that they are safe for everyone. The lack of FDA regulation means that supplements may contain little or none of the listed ingredients, and there is no long-term evidence of their safety and effectiveness. Some supplements can interact with other medications you may be taking, so tell your doctor if you plan to take glucosamine, chondroitin, or SAM-e, and report any side effects immediately.

procedure provides an alternative to joint replacement for people with arthritis whose bones are not strong enough to support a prosthesis or who have frequent joint infections that preclude the use of a prosthesis. Arthrodesis may also be used in small joints, such as the thumb, where replacements are performed less often.

Osteotomy and hemicallotasis. Osteotomy and hemicallotasis are procedures used to realign bones. For example, in the case of severely bowed legs that place excessive stress on the inner part of the knee joint, realignment of bone permits a more even distribution of weight across the joint. These procedure can be good options for more active people who wish to continue high-impact activities, such as skiing, which would cause a prosthetic joint to deteriorate and loosen.

In osteotomy, a wedge of bone in the knee or spine is cut away and the remaining bones are realigned. An osteotomy requires a hospital stay and a long recovery period but provides good relief of pain. Recovery is 80% complete in about six weeks and 100% complete within six months. About 1% of people who undergo osteotomy of the knee experience a complication called foot drop, in which the muscles on top of the foot become weakened or paralyzed as a result of nerve damage.

In hemicallotasis, the bone is realigned by lengthening it on one side. This is done by cutting the bone and attaching an external fixation device to the bone with pins. The patient turns screws on the device to slowly increase the distance between the cut ends of bone. The body sends new bone to the area, allowing the bone to lengthen about 1 mm a day. The fixation device must remain for about 12 weeks. The most serious complication of the device is infection where the pins enter the body.

Alternative and Complementary Treatments

The American College of Rheumatology reports that the data are "insufficient or inadequate" to sanction the use of pulsed electromagnetic fields, lasers, or vitamins and other dietary supplements for OA treatment. And while the National Institutes of Health is currently investigating glucosamine, chondroitin sulfate, and acupuncture in OA treatment, the American College of Rheumatology says it is "premature" to recommend their use. Nonetheless, glucosamine and chondroitin sulfate have received considerable media attention. For more information on these and other supplements for arthritis, see the feature on pages 24–25.

Treatments Under Development

To date, treatments for OA have provided symptom relief only and do not prevent or repair the underlying damage to the joint. Researchers are investigating new methods that may halt or actually repair the damage done by OA.

Human studies are under way on a new class of medications called disease-modifying osteoarthritis drugs (DMOADs). Since much of the damage from OA is thought to result from a disturbance in the natural cycle of cartilage destruction and rebuilding, DMOADs may eventually offer relief by inhibiting the release of enzymes that break down cartilage. Gene therapy is another new option being examined as a treatment for OA.

Rheumatoid Arthritis

Less common than osteoarthritis, rheumatoid arthritis (RA) affects 1% to 2% of the population (about 2.1 million people) and three times more women than men. The disease strikes multiple joints as well as other tissues and organs throughout the body. Although symptoms begin most often between ages 20 and 40, RA may develop at any age.

RA is an autoimmune disorder. Such disorders result when the body initiates an immune response against some natural body constituent mistakenly recognized as foreign. The joint damage caused by RA begins with inflammation of the synovial membrane that lines the joint. The inflammation leads to a thickening of the synovial membrane (pannus) due to overgrowth of synovial cells and accumulation of white blood cells. Release of enzymes and growth factors by the white blood cells, along with continuing growth of the pannus, can erode cartilage as well as bones, tendons, and ligaments within the joint capsule. As RA progresses, the production of excess tissue can further limit joint motion. Inflammation of tissues surrounding the joint also contributes to joint damage.

CAUSES OF RHEUMATOID ARTHRITIS

The exact cause of RA is unknown. Genetics play some role, since certain people inherit a susceptibility to the disease. There may also be an environmental factor that triggers RA, such as a virus or bacterium. Some studies have linked RA with cigarette smoking. A 2002 study found that the rate of new cases of arthritis has decreased steadily over the last 40 years, lending support to the hypothesis that a changing environmental factor may promote or protect against RA. For example, it is possible that birth control pills or hormone replacement therapy might offer some protection against RA, although not all studies have borne out this theory.

SYMPTOMS OF RHEUMATOID ARTHRITIS

Most often the onset of RA is marked by fatigue, weakness, low-grade fever, or loss of appetite and weight. Such symptoms may or may not be accompanied by mild joint stiffness or pain. When present, stiffness is most prominent in the morning and improves during the day. The period of stiffness lengthens when the disease is more active and tends to increase after strenuous activity.

The joints that most often become inflamed (red, warm, swollen, and painful) are those of the finger, wrist, knee, ankle, or toe—typically on both sides of the body. This symmetric pattern and the signs of inflammation distinguish RA from OA. Also, unlike OA, the joints

NEW RESEARCH

Antioxidant and Zinc May Reduce Risk of RA

Eating a diet rich in the antioxidant beta-cryptoxanthin and taking zinc supplements may reduce the risk of developing rheumatoid arthritis (RA), according to preliminary research.

Previous studies have suggested that antioxidants may offer some protection against RA, but this research is the first to look specifically at beta-cryptoxanthin, a carotenoid found in foods such as oranges and grapefruit juice. It is also the first study to evaluate the role of zinc in the development of RA.

The study included nearly 30,000 women (age 55 to 69) who filled out dietary questionnaires in 1986 as part of the Iowa Women's Health Study. When the women were contacted up to eleven years later, 152 of them had been diagnosed with RA.

Women with the highest dietary intake of beta-cryptoxanthin were 41% less likely to develop RA than those with the lowest intake. Those who took at least 15 mg a day of zinc supplements were 61% less likely to develop RA than those who did not take supplemental zinc.

Antioxidants such as beta-cryptoxanthin are hypothesized to protect against tissue damage in RA, while zinc plays a role in immune function. But until more is known, doctors do not recommend any dietary measures to prevent RA.

AMERICAN JOURNAL OF EPIDEMIOLOGY
Volume 157, page 345
February 15, 2003

Traveling With Arthritis

People with arthritis often find traveling difficult. But you can take measures to minimize stiffness and pain, regardless of the mode of transportation.

Traveling can be a great way to relax or spend time with family. But for people with arthritis, getting to and from their destination can be more stressful than their regular routine. Sitting for long periods may make joints stiff, and dealing with luggage, transfers, and cramped seating can all contribute to pain and fatigue. Fortunately, whether you travel by plane, train, bus, car, or cruise ship, there are ways to minimize stress on joints.

Plane

Tips for traveling by plane:

Planning. It's important to make reservations early so that you will have more options. Be sure to mention any special needs to the reservation agent. Try to book a non-stop, direct flight to eliminate transfers, and avoid traveling at peak times of the day. Ask for a seat in an exit row or the bulkhead; these seats have more leg room. If you will need assistance in getting around the terminal, request a wheelchair or an airport cart in advance.

En route. Check your large luggage so you won't end up carrying it. Carry your medications on board with you, in case your checked baggage gets lost or delayed. Also, take copies of your prescriptions and your doctor's telephone number to minimize hassles when going through security. Bring along healthy snacks, and be sure to drink enough water to prevent dehydration. Use the small airline pillows to support your back or neck. Inform the flight attendant that you have arthritis and that you may need to get up periodically to stretch during the flight. Try the stretching exercises in the inset box on the opposite page to prevent joint stiffness.

Train

Tips for traveling by train:

Planning. Make reservations early to guarantee a seat. Ask about discounted fares for disabled passengers. If needed, reserve a wheelchair at your stop and find out whether porters will be available to help you with boarding and exiting. Special requests can be made through Amtrak's special service desk.

En route. Be sure to pack lightly if you think you may be unable to get assistance with getting your baggage on and off the train. Remember to bring your own snacks so that you won't need to walk through the train to the dining car. Try to obtain an aisle seat near the restroom. Get up periodically and do the stretching exercises described in the inset box on the opposite page.

Bus

Tips for traveling by bus:

Planning. Consider scheduling trips for weekdays, when fewer people travel and buses are less crowded. Try to book your trip with as few

at the tips of the fingers are generally not affected by RA. Another characteristic feature of RA is the formation of hard bumps under the skin, called rheumatoid nodules. Rheumatoid nodules can be found in tissues throughout the body, especially around the joints. About 20% of people with RA have rheumatoid nodules.

In active RA, the joints are inflamed and progressive joint damage occurs. Active RA may include periods of worsening inflammation called flare-ups, or flares. Joint damage stops only when the disease is controlled with medication. Occasionally, the disease goes into remission and medications can be discontinued.

RA can lead to additional health problems. Approximately one third of people with RA develop mild anemia, a decreased number of red blood cells. About 10% to 15% of people with RA (mostly women) develop Sjögren's syndrome, a chronic condition that leads to dry eyes and mouth. RA can also lead to inflammation of transfers as possible. If you travel with an aide, a two-for-one fare may be available. Since most bus aisles are not wide enough to accommodate a wheelchair, ask customer service if assistance will be available for getting on and off the bus. Also ask if a wheelchair must be collapsible to be transported on the bus.

En route. Bring a pillow or a cervical collar to make naps more comfortable. Take along snacks or small meals if you anticipate that it will be difficult to get off the bus at food stops. Try the stretching exercises in the inset box at right to avoid stiffness.

Car

Tips for traveling by car:

Planning. Traveling by car offers the most freedom, as you can set your own schedule and stop whenever you like. Still, it's important to plan for contingencies. Remember to take a handicapped parking permit with you, if you have one. Also, bring medications, snacks, maps, and water and pack them in easily accessible places. Consider taking along a cell phone. When renting a car, ask

---

Maintaining Good Posture and Flexibility

Good posture is important during travel to keep stiffness and pain at bay. Sit up straight, pull in your stomach muscles, and keep your shoulders down and relaxed. To help maintain this posture while driving, keep the rearview mirror at a level that forces you to sit up tall. In addition, the following stretching exercises can help minimize stiffness:

• Raise and lower your shoulders a few times, and then rotate them in circles.
• Tilt your head gently to the right and then to the left; then turn your head slowly to each side.
• Stretch your arms in front of you, then out to the side, and finally toward your back, squeezing your shoulder blades together.
• Make a fist with both hands; then open your hands and separate your fingers as far apart as you can.
• Rotate your ankles, then flex them a few times.

---

about special features, such as power steering, cruise control, and lift-up door handles.

En route. Riding in a car for extended periods can lead to joint stiffness and swelling. To prevent this, stop about every hour and a half and do the stretching exercises described in the inset box above.

Cruise Ship

Tips for taking a cruise:

Planning. Before booking a cruise, ask about the ship's design and accessibility, such as whether hallways, doorways, and elevators are wide enough for a wheelchair and whether rooms are wheelchair accessible. Also mention any special dietary needs when making your reservation.

En route. Some cruise ships offer gentle exercise classes, which you may wish to try to help minimize joint stiffness. If disembarking at stops is difficult, you may wish to stay on board while others go ashore.

---

the white outer layer of the eye (scleritis) or the membrane lining the chest (pleurisy). Rarely, it can cause inflammation of the blood vessels (vasculitis) or the membrane surrounding the heart (pericarditis). Nerve damage (neuropathy) may occur when an inflamed joint compresses a nerve. An extremely rare complication of RA called Felty Syndrome involves an enlarged spleen and a low white blood cell count, causing recurrent infections.

DIAGNOSIS OF RHEUMATOID ARTHRITIS

RA is difficult to diagnose in its early stages, when the joints may appear normal. Initially, the diagnosis is made by ruling out other possible causes for the symptoms. The doctor will take a medical history and conduct a physical examination similar to the one used to diagnose osteoarthritis (see pages 5–6). The presence of RA can be confirmed later with x-rays and laboratory tests.

Certainly, the finding of multiple red, swollen joints that are warm to the touch is strongly suggestive of RA, particularly if the same joints are involved on both sides of the body. However, these signs are present only during the active stages of the disease and may not be detectable in joints such as the hip that are deeply buried in the body.

Medical History

For the best treatment, patients must honestly answer their doctors' questions about pain, disability, limitations in activity, fatigue, and other symptoms. In addition, people should not hesitate to mention any symptoms that the doctor did not ask about. Although this advice may seem obvious, a recent study found that women with RA tended to downplay the severity of their symptoms when consulting doctors. Since doctors rely on people's reports of pain, stiffness, disability, and other symptoms in choosing among therapeutic options, stoic responses may adversely affect the quality of treatment.

Laboratory Tests

The diagnosis of RA can be made more certain by documenting the presence of synovitis—inflammation of the synovial membrane. Synovitis can be detected by withdrawing a small amount of fluid from the joint and counting the number of white blood cells, which fight infection but can also cause inflammation. Other causes of synovitis must still be considered, however. Although x-rays of affected joints are not useful during the early stages of RA, those taken more than six months after the onset of active disease can show the characteristic narrowing of the joint space and the bony erosions that point to a diagnosis of RA.

A blood test to check for the presence of rheumatoid factor is also useful. Rheumatoid factor is an abnormal protein present in the blood of about 85% of people with RA; larger amounts of this protein are present when the disease is most severe. Many people with RA who initially test negative for rheumatoid factor will test positive as the disease progresses. However, this test is not definitive because elevated levels of rheumatoid factor can be found in people with other autoimmune diseases, as well as a number of unrelated disorders. Other common blood abnormalities indicative of RA are mild anemia, an elevated sedimentation rate (a nonspecific sign of inflammation), and a low white blood cell count.

Prognosis

About 10% of people diagnosed with RA experience long-term remission within one year. Another 40% to 65% go into remission within two years. In these two groups of patients, rheumatoid factor levels often are low or absent, and symptoms are relatively mild, even when the disease is active. The prognosis is much worse if the disease remains active for more than two years. Such patients have a far greater chance of significant joint deformity.

If the disease progresses for months or years, affected joints eventually become deformed and their range of motion is increasingly limited. The muscles may become atrophied from lack of use. Other possible side effects are carpal tunnel syndrome (pain, numbness, or tingling in the hand) and dryness of the eyes, mouth, and other mucous membranes. Less frequently, people may experience more serious systemic problems (problems affecting other sites in the body). These include an enlarged spleen and inflammation of the heart, the membrane covering the heart (pericarditis), the membranes surrounding the lungs (pleurisy), and the outer layers of the eyes (which can lead to blindness).

People with RA have a shorter life span than the general population, largely owing to an increased risk of heart disease. This increase might be explained by the fact that people with RA tend to exercise less. It is also possible that the inflammation characteristic of RA contributes to the high rate of heart disease. In recent years, researchers have found that inflammation accelerates the buildup of atherosclerotic plaque in arteries.

For this reason, people with RA need to take extra steps to prevent heart disease, such as eating a diet low in fat and cholesterol and exercising several times a week (physical activity can help with arthritis symptoms as well). Because high blood cholesterol levels and high blood pressure increase the risk of heart disease, people with RA may need to take medications to lower their blood cholesterol levels and blood pressure.

TREATMENT OF RHEUMATOID ARTHRITIS

The goals in the treatment of RA are to relieve pain, reduce inflammation, maintain function, and prevent joint deformities. Medications are required to control pain and diminish inflammation. Other components of therapy include an appropriate mixture of rest and gentle exercise, as well as physical therapy and protection of the joints. A thorough understanding of the disease and a positive

NEW RESEARCH

Rheumatoid Arthritis Impairs Function More in Women

Treatment of rheumatoid arthritis (RA) is aimed at controlling symptoms and maintaining functional abilities. But a new study shows that even when the disease is well managed, functional abilities are impaired in the long run—especially in women.

Swedish researchers followed 196 women and 88 men with RA for two years. All patients received appropriate treatment, such as analgesics, nonsteroidal anti-inflammatory drugs, disease-modifying antirheumatic drugs, or corticosteroids. At regular intervals, patients were evaluated for disease severity based on various symptoms—including pain, tenderness, and morning stiffness—and laboratory tests. The researchers also measured functional abilities, such as hand function, range of movement, and the amount of time needed to walk a predetermined distance.

During the first three months, both disease severity and functional abilities improved equally for men and women, then stayed constant for about a year. During the second year, disease severity remained stable but there was a general decline in functional abilities, especially in women.

The authors concluded that function can deteriorate even when the disease activity of RA is effectively treated.

ANNALS OF RHEUMATIC DISEASES
Volume 62, page 667
July 2003

attitude are also important. One recent change in the standard approach to treating RA is a movement among physicians to prescribe stronger antirheumatic drugs (see pages 36–44) earlier in the course of the disease, in an effort to control symptoms more quickly and minimize joint damage.

People with RA can benefit from many of the treatments used for OA (see page 7): application of ice to affected joints to reduce pain and inflammation, exercise to build strength and flexibility, and surgery to replace damaged joints. Topical products, however, are not helpful in RA. Additional medications may be needed to control inflammation. People with RA also must pay special attention to combating fatigue, which can be the most incapacitating feature of the disease.

Developing strategies to cope with the emotional and psychological factors associated with RA is also a key part of treatment that should not be overlooked. People with arthritis have especially high rates of depression. About 20% of people with RA are depressed, compared with 2% to 3% of men and 5% to 9% of women in the general population.

Rest

Proper rest when joints are inflamed can help relieve fatigue. Complete bed rest may be necessary during periods of severe inflammation involving multiple joints. People with RA need about 10 hours of sleep a day, either all at night or about 8 hours at night and 2 hours during daytime naps. Napping during the day should be avoided if it interferes with nighttime sleep, however. For more information about coping with the fatigue of arthritis, see the feature on the opposite page.

When inflammation is present—but not severe enough to require complete bed rest—joints should be rested properly to avoid flexion contracture. Flexion contracture is a loss of joint motion due to shortening of the surrounding tissues, especially in the hips and knees. Listed below are three tips for proper resting technique:

- Do not remain seated for a long time; be sure to stand up periodically.
- If weight-bearing joints such as the hips or knees are affected, protect them by using crutches or braces when starting to walk again after a period of severe inflammation.
- Apply removable splints (see below) to inflamed joints to alleviate muscle spasm and diminish the likelihood of deformities.

Coping With the Fatigue of Arthritis

Getting enough rest can help control your pain—and pain control can help you get a good night's sleep.

People with arthritis often find that fatigue, not pain, is the most debilitating symptom of their condition. Fatigue can cause a person to feel devoid of energy, moody, irritable, and unable to concentrate.

Fatigue associated with autoimmune disorders such as rheumatoid arthritis and lupus may have a variety of causes. These include chronic inflammation, a flare in symptoms, or anemia (low red blood cell count). One theory holds that inflammatory cytokines—substances produced during times of acute or chronic illness—cause fatigue and may be the body's way of telling you to get more rest to help you recover.

Additional factors can lead to fatigue in people with arthritis. These include sleeping poorly due to pain, feeling depressed, or favoring a healthy joint over an arthritic one, which can quickly tire you out by placing unusual strain on your muscles and tendons.

Finally, fatigue can be a self-perpetuating problem: People who feel fatigued may drink caffeine or take daytime naps, which lead to poor nighttime sleep and further fatigue. Being tired can also make people avoid exercise, producing muscle weakness and more fatigue. However, there are effective ways to decrease your fatigue and to cope with its effects at times when it is unavoidable.

How To Reduce Fatigue

A few small changes could help restore some of your lost energy:

Keep pain under control. Pain contributes to fatigue, so try to decrease it as much as possible with ice packs, heat, rest, or medications. Talk to your doctor about the most effective ways to minimize your pain.

Get enough sleep. People with rheumatoid arthritis need about 10 hours of sleep a night. People with lupus need between 8 and 10 hours of sleep a night.

Improve your sleep habits. If you are having trouble sleeping at night, avoid naps during the day. Also, avoid caffeine and alcohol before bedtime, keep your bedroom dark and cool, and take a warm bath at night to relax your muscles.

Be more active. Rest is important when your body needs it, but try to stay as active as possible. Physical activity will help you sleep better at night and stay in better shape; both can help ward off fatigue.

Listen to your body. Fatigue could be a sign that you are working too hard or pushing yourself beyond your limits. When your body tells you that you need to rest, listen to it.

How To Live With Fatigue

If fatigue is still a problem after taking the above steps, you may need to make some adjustments to your everyday activities.

Prioritize. When fatigue is especially bad, tackle only the tasks that are absolutely necessary.

Be organized. A little advance planning can save you a lot of energy—for example, rearrange your kitchen so that frequently used items are within easy reach.

Pace yourself. Breaking down a large task into several smaller ones can make it more manageable. For example, instead of trying to vacuum the whole house at once, try doing one room in the morning and another in the afternoon.

Be flexible. Let friends and family know that you have limitations and that you might need to cancel plans if you are not feeling well. Make sure you give yourself a break, too—it is perfectly acceptable to heat up frozen dinners on days when you do not feel up to cooking.

Find a support group. Other people with arthritis can be a valuable resource for more coping strategies and ways to reduce fatigue. To locate a support group in your area, contact the Arthritis Foundation (see page 76 for contact information).

Braces, Splints, and Assistive Devices

Braces and splints are over-the-counter or custom-made supports designed to relieve pain and stabilize and protect joints during periods of inflammation, when joints (especially those in the hands and wrists) are more prone to injury. Splints should be lightweight and easy to remove, allowing for range-of-motion exercises several times daily. Prolonged or improper use of splints can increase stiffness and progressively diminish muscle strength and joint mobility.

Splints are most effective for the hands, wrists, or both. The best "splint" for the hip and knee joints is lying in a face-down position on a firm bed for about 15 minutes several times a day. Long-term use of splints for the elbow and shoulder joints poses the risk of rapid loss of mobility in these joints. As a result, judicious use of local treatments such as injections of inflammation-reducing steroids and appropriate use of physical therapy are preferable.

Assistive devices (such as faucet turners or jar openers) help decrease the difficulty of everyday tasks. Occupational therapists are experts in fitting braces and splints, recommending assistive devices, and instructing patients on their proper use.

Exercise

When joints are inflamed, only gentle exercises such as bending and straightening the joint are appropriate. Resistance exercises, which may involve light weights or working against the body's own weight, can be introduced gradually as joint inflammation subsides. However, any exercise that causes worsened pain an hour later should be avoided. When joints are not inflamed, moderate aerobic exercises should be performed to help increase endurance and keep joints flexible.

Aquatic exercise is an especially good exercise option for people with RA. Like other forms of exercise, it can increase joint flexibility, strengthen muscles, provide a good aerobic workout, and boost self-confidence. But aquatic workouts offer several additional advantages. Because water supports much of the body's weight, exercise in a pool allows people with arthritis to move about with minimal stress on their joints. For people with impaired balance, it also eliminates the risk of falling while exercising. In addition, warm water itself is therapeutic and can provide significant pain relief. The Arthritis Foundation can recommend aquatic therapy programs and offer instructional videotapes.

Drug Treatment: Nonsteroidal Anti-Inflammatory Drugs

Unless there is some reason not to use aspirin, such as an allergy, this medication is usually the first treatment attempted for RA. Aspirin is effective in reducing inflammation and is less expensive than the other NSAIDs. The dosage depends on a balance between the large amounts of aspirin that may be needed to control symptoms and the development of side effects. (For more on NSAIDs, see pages 13–18 and the chart on pages 16–17.)

Other NSAIDs, including the newer class of drugs called the

Easing Foot, Ankle, and Knee Pain With Orthotics

These special shoe inserts can reduce pain and improve function in the lower body, primarily by redistributing weight or absorbing shock.

The feet each have 33 joints and are highly susceptible to osteoarthritis (OA), rheumatoid arthritis (RA), and other painful conditions. Foot discomfort and deformity caused by these conditions can even lead to pain in the shins, knees, and lower back.

One way to minimize problems caused by arthritis in the feet or ankles is to correct misalignments and poor biomechanics in the feet with shoe inserts; the result is reduced stress on joints in the feet, ankles, and knees and less lower body discomfort and deformity caused by OA or RA (particularly in the early stages of these conditions). While some people may benefit from over-the-counter shoe inserts, others require custom-made orthoses (often called orthotics).

Orthotics work in several ways. First, by distributing weight more evenly over the bottom of the foot, they reduce pressure on sore or sensitive areas. Second, certain orthotics contain shock-absorbing material to lessen the stress placed on the lower body when walking or running. Third, orthotics may compensate for structural or biomechanical abnormalities in the feet or ankles. Lastly, orthotics can reduce wear and tear on joints by limiting their motion.

Types of Orthotics
There are two basic types of orthotics: accommodative and functional. Accommodative orthotics are the softer variety and are typically made from materials like plastic foam, rubber, cork, or leather. They are designed to cushion tender feet and are often used by patients with diabetic ulcers, calluses, or soreness on the soles of the feet.

Functional orthotics are made of more rigid material—such as thermoplastic polymers, acrylic plastic, or graphite—and are more likely to be used by patients with pain in the toes, arches, heels, or ankles, or discomfort in the knee and hip caused by poor biomechanics in the foot and ankle. These more rigid orthotics can also help people with shin splints and those with bursitis or tendinitis in the lower body.

Orthotics can be made with both an accommodative and a functional design, and they are often individualized to address a patient's specific problem. Most people with arthritis require orthotics that have both accommodative and functional properties.

Making the Orthotic
To obtain orthotics, you first must be examined by a podiatrist. The podiatrist will likely examine your feet, ankles, knees, and hips while you are sitting and standing. He or she may also take measurements and observe how your lower body works while you walk.

If the podiatrist feels you could benefit from orthotics, a three-dimensional model of the bottom of your feet will be made. This can be done either by having you place your bare feet in a plaster cast or by using computerized scanning techniques to create an image of your feet. Typically, the podiatrist sends the model of your feet to a laboratory, along with a prescription that describes the modifications that need to be made to address your specific problems.

Custom-made orthotics can cost around $450 per pair. Some health insurance plans cover the cost of prescription orthotics, but many do not. If you are unable to pay for a pair of custom-made orthotics, a podiatrist may be able to modify over-the-counter inserts to fit your needs.

Wearing Your Orthotics
Although orthotics are custom designed for your feet, they may feel uncomfortable at first. Experts suggest that you begin by wearing them for a half hour to two hours a day and then lengthen the time you wear them by 45 minutes each day. The orthotics should be adjusted if they cause pain or leave indentations on your feet. Orthotics tend to fit better in shoes with removable insoles, since the orthotics take up extra room in your shoes. When you shop for shoes, be sure to have your orthotics with you so you can purchase footwear that can accommodate them. A quality pair of functional orthotics can last about five years.

COX-2 inhibitors, are employed when aspirin is ineffective or causes serious side effects. These drugs are more expensive than aspirin, but compliance may be better because they are taken fewer times each day. In addition, some (but not all) studies suggest that COX-2 inhibitors have fewer gastrointestinal side effects than other NSAIDs, although some people respond better to one drug than another.

As in the treatment of OA, the goal is to use the NSAID that provides the greatest benefit while producing the fewest side effects; some trial and error may be needed.

Drug Treatment: Antirheumatics

The current trend is to start using potent antirheumatic drugs right away if basic anti-inflammatories fail to control symptoms. These potent drugs (see the chart on pages 38–39) are usually referred to as disease-modifying antirheumatic drugs (DMARDs) but are also called SAARDs (slow-acting antirheumatic drugs).

Antimalarials. The most commonly used antimalarial is hydroxychloroquine (Plaquenil). Between 30% and 40% of people with RA respond to this drug, but improvement does not begin for three to six months. A typical dosage is 200 mg twice a day. The advantage of this drug is its low incidence of side effects. The most serious risk—vision loss due to damage to the retina—is rare at low dosages, but regular eye exams are required during long-term treatment. Other side effects are gastrointestinal problems and, in rare instances, inflammation of the nervous system and skeletal and heart muscles.

Azathioprine. Azathioprine (Imuran) is an antimetabolite (a substance that blocks a normal metabolic process) and is most commonly employed as an immunosuppressant to prevent rejection of transplanted kidneys and hearts. The dosage depends on body weight but usually ranges from 50 to 150 mg a day. Azathioprine's mechanism of action in RA is unknown. In addition, the drug can take two or three months to work. Because it can cause dangerous suppression of the immune system that may lead to serious infection, it is used only when severe symptoms fail to respond to safer drugs. Digestive side effects, such as loss of appetite, nausea, or, rarely, vomiting, may develop.

Corticosteroids. The corticosteroid drug prednisone (Deltasone, Meticorten, Prednisone Intensol, Sterapred) usually produces rapid and dramatic symptomatic improvement by reducing inflammation and suppressing the immune system, but disease manifestations frequently recur once the steroid is discontinued. As a result, physicians and patients alike have been tempted to continue steroid use for long periods, despite many serious side effects that mimic Cushing's disease, a disorder caused by overproduction of corticosteroids by the adrenal glands.

Side effects of long-term corticosteroid treatment include stomach ulcers, weight gain with fat deposits in the trunk of the body (especially in the upper back), diabetes, high blood pressure, thinning of the skin with easy bruising and poor wound healing, acne, weakness, muscle wasting, cataracts, increased susceptibility to infections, and psychiatric disturbances.

Because osteoporosis is also an important side effect of steroid use, occurring in as many as 50% of patients, the American College of Rheumatology has developed guidelines to help prevent a decrease in bone density in people using corticosteroids. In general, the American College of Rheumatology recommends that the lowest effective dose of steroid be used and that people adhere to such lifestyle measures as not smoking, maintaining a healthy weight, and limiting alcohol consumption. A baseline bone scan should be done before beginning therapy for comparison purposes. Follow-up scans every six months to one year afterward can be used to monitor changes in bone density. Also, people taking steroids should get 1,500 mg of calcium and 400 to 800 IU of vitamin D daily.

Low-dose hormone replacement therapy can be used to maintain or improve bone density in postmenopausal women, but this treatment has been associated with a small increase in the risk of breast cancer and cardiovascular disease. For this reason, an osteoporosis treatment such as alendronate (Fosamax), risedronate (Actonel), or calcitonin (Calcimar, Miacalcin) may be a better choice.

Corticosteroid use is best reserved for the acute treatment of incapacitating flares of joint disease, for severe manifestations of RA affecting other organs, or when alternative drugs are unsuccessful or cause intolerable side effects.

When corticosteroids are discontinued after being used at high doses or for a long time, the dose must be reduced very slowly. This is done to allow the adrenal glands to resume production of steroids (the adrenal glands stop producing steroids during corticosteroid administration) and to help prevent a flare of arthritis.

Cyclophosphamide. The anticancer drug cyclophosphamide (Cytoxan, Neosar) has proven beneficial in studies of people with RA who have not responded adequately to any other therapeutic measures. People taking this drug must drink plenty of fluids to maintain good urine flow, since serious inflammation of the bladder (hemorrhagic cystitis) is a possible side effect. Cyclophosphamide can cause fetal damage if administered to a pregnant woman, an important concern because many RA sufferers are women of childbearing age. The correct dosage is based on a number of factors, including body weight.

Cyclosporine. The drug cyclosporine (Neoral, Sandimmune) is

NEW RESEARCH

Body Weight Linked to Osteoporosis in People With RA

Rheumatoid arthritis (RA) appears to be linked to an increased risk of osteoporosis. Now, a Swedish study suggests that the risk of osteoporosis in women with RA is greatest among those with low body weight and extensive joint damage.

Researchers evaluated bone mineral density and joint damage in 88 postmenopausal women with RA. None of the women were taking bisphosphonates or hormone replacement therapy, both of which can slow the rate of bone loss.

Forty-eight percent of the women had osteoporosis in the femoral neck (part of the hip joint), compared with 7% of healthy Swedish women in the same age group. Low body weight was the strongest risk factor for osteoporosis: Women with osteoporosis weighed an average of 22 lbs. less than women with normal bone mineral density and had more extensive joint damage. Other factors associated with bone loss included advancing age, duration of RA, functional disabilities, and regular treatment with corticosteroid medications.

The reason for the association between low body weight and increased joint damage is unclear, but the researchers say future studies should examine whether aggressive treatment of RA to prevent joint damage can help protect bone density as well.

ANNALS OF RHEUMATIC DISEASES
Volume 62, page 617
July 2003

Commonly Used Disease-Modifying Antirheumatic Drugs 2004

Generic Name	Brand Name	Average Dosage*	Wholesale Cost (Generic Cost)†
adalimumab	Humira	40 mg every other week	40 mg vial: $653
anakinra	Kineret	100 mg/day	100 mg syringe: $44
azathioprine	Imuran	50 to 150 mg/day	50 mg: $222 ($131)
cyclophosphamide	Cytoxan Neosar	1 to 3 mg/kg/day	50 mg: $432 ($373) 100 mg of powder: $6
cyclosporine	Neoral Sandimmune	2.5 to 4 mg/kg/day	100 mg: $611 ($574) 100 mg: $693 ($574)
etanercept	Enbrel	25 mg twice a week	25 mg vial: $163
gold salts, oral: auranofin	Ridaura	3 mg twice a day	3 mg: $305
gold salts, injectable: gold sodium thiomalate	Myochrysine	25 to 50 mg maintenance dose every two to four weeks	50 mg/mL, 10 mL: $118

* These dosages represent an average range for the treatment of rheumatoid arthritis (RA). The precise effective dosage varies from patient to patient and depends on many factors. Do not make any changes in your medication without consulting your doctor. Milligrams per kilogram of body weight per day is represented as mg/kg/day.

† Average wholesale prices to pharmacists for 100 tablets or capsules (unless otherwise indicated) of the dosage strength listed. Costs to consumers are higher. If a generic version is available, the cost is listed in parentheses. Source: Red Book, 2003 (Medical Economics Data, publishers).

How They Work	Comments
Inhibits the activity of a protein called tumor necrosis factor that invades the joints of people with RA. Can delay structural damage in people with moderate to severe RA.	The drug must be injected every other week under the skin, and the site of the shot should be rotated regularly. Common side effects are irritation at the injection site, sinus infections, headache, and nausea. Rare side effects are serious infections (including tuberculosis), nervous system diseases, cancer, lupus-like symptoms, and allergic reactions.
Inhibits the activity of a protein called interleukin-1 that invades the joints of people with RA. Must be injected once a day; takes about one month to be effective.	Most people experience redness, swelling, bruising, itching, or stinging at the injection site. Applying a cold pack on the injection site immediately after injection can minimize swelling and bruising. Increases the chance of developing a serious infection, so tell your doctor right away if you develop an infection that does not go away while taking the drug. Periodic tests are required to check white blood cell count.
Inhibits the abnormal immune response leading to RA. May take two to three months to be effective.	Only used when severe symptoms fail to respond to safer drugs, since it increases susceptibility to infection and abnormal bleeding. Side effects include nausea, vomiting, appetite loss, and, less commonly, liver problems, skin rash, and mouth sores. Taking doses right after meals reduces stomach irritation. Do not use during pregnancy or breast-feeding. Avoid alcohol. Seek medical attention for fever or bleeding.
An anticancer drug. Relieves RA symptoms through an unknown mechanism.	Side effects include nausea, vomiting, loss of appetite and weight, temporary hair loss, skin rash, increased pigmentation in skin and fingernails, ringing in the ears or hearing loss, temporary or sometimes permanent sterility in men, fatigue, dizziness, confusion, and susceptibility to infection. Avoid the drug during pregnancy. Take on an empty stomach (or with small amounts of food or milk to prevent stomach irritation), and drink plenty of fluids to prevent bladder inflammation and bleeding, a rare but serious side effect.
Inhibits the activity of white blood cells, a key participant in RA joint inflammation.	May cause kidney damage and high blood pressure; patients should be monitored for these problems throughout treatment. More common side effects include headache, tremor, unusual hair growth on the body and face, swelling or bleeding of the gums, increased susceptibility to infection, and increased skin sensitivity to sunlight. Take with food to minimize stomach irritation. Avoid alcohol and maintain good dental hygiene, since cyclosporine can cause gum problems.
Inhibits the activity of a protein called tumor necrosis factor that invades the joints of people with RA. Can delay structural damage in people with moderate to severe RA.	The drug must be injected twice a week under the skin, and the site of the shot should be rotated regularly. With a doctor's approval, patients can be taught to inject the medication themselves. Serious infections, low blood counts, and worsening of heart failure have been reported in people using etanercept. Patients should be monitored for confusion, numbness, changes in vision, and difficulty walking, which may suggest a rare but serious condition called demyelination. Common side effects are irritation at the injection site, headache, and allergic reactions.
These agents reduce the painful joint inflammation of active RA. Usually take effect in three to six months.	Given by either injection or pills. Possible side effects include skin rash, inflammation of the mucous membranes in the mouth (stomatitis), diarrhea (more common with oral gold), kidney damage, appetite loss, nausea and vomiting, indigestion, constipation, itching, and temporary joint pain shortly after an injection. To reduce diarrhea, eat a diet high in fiber and begin oral gold with low doses that are increased slowly. Periodic blood and urine tests are necessary to check for anemia, low white blood cell count, or protein in the urine. Avoid alcohol.

Commonly Used Disease-Modifying Antirheumatic Drugs 2004 (continued)

Generic Name	Brand Name	Average Dosage*	Wholesale Cost (Generic Cost)†
hydroxychloroquine	Plaquenil	200 mg twice a day	200 mg: $175 ($113)
infliximab	Remicade	3 to 10 mg every eight weeks	100 mg vial: $692
leflunomide	Arava	100 mg/day for the first three days, followed by 10 to 20 mg/day	20 mg: $1012
methotrexate	Rheumatrex	7.5 to 20 mg/week	2.5 mg: $497 ($336)
minocycline	Dynacin Minocin	100 mg twice a day	100 mg: $467 ($287) 100 mg: $389 ($287)
penicillamine	Cuprimine Depen	250 to 750 mg/day	250 mg: $116 250 mg: $295
prednisone	Deltasone Prednisone Intensol Sterapred Prednicot	5 to 250 mg/day	10 mg: $7 ($10) 5 mg/mL, 30 mL: $31 5 mg: $43 10 mg: $4 ($10)
sulfasalazine	Azulfidine EN-tabs	1,000 mg two to three times a day	500 mg: $45 ($25)

* These dosages represent an average range for the treatment of RA. The precise effective dosage varies from patient to patient and depends on many factors. Do not make any changes in your medication without consulting your doctor.

† Average wholesale prices to pharmacists for 100 tablets or capsules (unless otherwise indicated) of the dosage strength listed. Costs to consumers are higher. If a generic version is available, the cost is listed in parentheses. Source: *Red Book, 2003* (Medical Economics Data, publishers).

How They Work	Comments
Normally used to treat malaria; may suppress the release of certain inflammatory substances. May take up to six months to be effective.	Side effects are uncommon but include diarrhea, appetite loss, headache, stomach pain or cramping, itching, and dizziness. People on long-term therapy should have eye exams twice a year to check for damage to the retina, a rare but serious side effect.
Originally approved for the treatment of Crohn's disease. Inhibits the activity of a protein called tumor necrosis factor that invades the joints of people with RA.	Administered in combination with methotrexate through an intravenous infusion, followed by additional infusions at two and six weeks and every eight weeks thereafter. Serious infections have been reported in people using infliximab; patients should be evaluated for latent tuberculosis, and tuberculosis infection should be treated before beginning therapy. Serious neurological problems also have been reported; people should be monitored for confusion, numbness, changes in vision, and difficulty walking. People with heart failure should not begin taking the drug. Other possible side effects are acute reactions to the infusion and headache.
Blocks the overproduction of immune cells that cause inflammation of the joints.	Side effects include liver toxicity, diarrhea, skin rash, and hair loss. Do not use during pregnancy or when attempting to become pregnant. Avoid the drug altogether if you have significant liver disease.
Appears to inhibit the abnormal immune response associated with RA. Once-a-week therapy can improve RA symptoms in one to two months.	Side effects include gastrointestinal bleeding, appetite loss, nausea, vomiting, mouth ulcers, skin sensitivity to sunlight, susceptibility to infection, acne, boils, and skin rash. Take doses one to two hours before a meal, avoid alcohol, and have blood tests every four to eight weeks to monitor liver function.
Unclear, but may work by reducing joint inflammation.	Side effects are uncommon but include upset stomach, itching of the rectum or vagina, diarrhea, dizziness or light-headedness, furry darkening or black discoloration of the tongue, rash, and sun sensitivity.
Unclear, but may work by suppressing the body's release of certain chemicals that cause inflammation. May take two to three months to work.	May cause diarrhea, nausea, vomiting, loss of taste, mild stomach pain, appetite loss, mouth ulcers, fever, rash, or low levels of platelets and white blood cells. Take on an empty stomach, and don't use during pregnancy. Avoid taking iron-containing supplements or medications within two hours of a dose, but take 25 mg of vitamin B_6 daily, since the drug increases the need for this vitamin. Blood and urine tests are needed every one to three months to check for a toxic reaction.
Inhibits the release and activity of inflammatory substances in the body and suppresses the immune system.	Can cause rapid, dramatic improvement of joint inflammation but should be used only for severe joint flares or serious nonjoint manifestations of RA because of the potential for side effects. Side effects include increased appetite, nervousness, cataracts, diabetes, high blood pressure, osteoporosis, stomach ulcers, weight gain, slow healing of wounds, easy bruising, acne, weakness, muscle wasting, and infection. Even at low doses, long-term use can cause symptoms of acute adrenal insufficiency. Long-term use should be ended slowly to prevent a flare of RA.
Reduces inflammation and suppresses the immune system. Usually takes effect in one to three months.	Side effects include abdominal cramps, diarrhea, appetite loss, nausea and vomiting, dizziness, rash, and headache. May also cause skin yellowing (jaundice) or sensitivity to the sun. Take pills with a full glass of water at meals to minimize gastrointestinal symptoms. Lower doses can also help.

an immunosuppressant that is most commonly used to prevent rejection of transplanted organs. It relieves symptoms of RA by inhibiting the growth and action of immune system cells, including those that cause joint pain and swelling. Because it is highly toxic and can cause high blood pressure and damage to the kidneys, it should be administered in low doses over a period of time, and patients must be monitored closely. The correct dosage is based on a number of factors, including body weight, but ranges from 2.5 to 4 g/kg a day.

Gold salts. Therapy with gold salts (chrysotherapy), which is used in people who do not respond to NSAIDs and are unable to take methotrexate (see below), is beneficial about 60% of the time. Gold salts appear to act by suppressing synovial inflammation during active RA. The benefits of treatment are not apparent for about three to six months. Gold is administered either by intramuscular injections or by oral dosages—though injected gold is more effective overall than oral treatment. The injections start at 10 mg a week, then range from 25 to 50 mg every two to four weeks. Initial oral dosages are about 3 mg twice a day.

Side effects, which occur in about a third of people receiving gold injections, include inflammation of the skin and mucous membranes of the mouth, protein in the urine, and a drop in white blood cell levels. Diarrhea (which can be reduced by high-fiber diets and by starting with low doses that are increased slowly) occurs more often with oral treatment; the other side effects, especially protein in the urine, occur more often with injections. About 4% to 5% of patients must stop gold therapy because of gastrointestinal side effects. Even those who have tolerated gold injections for several years need to watch for adverse reactions, including dizziness, nausea, and pain within an hour of the injection. Regular blood tests are necessary to monitor side effects.

Methotrexate. Methotrexate (Rheumatrex), which acts as a mild immunosuppressant, was first used to treat some forms of cancer. It is now recognized as the drug of choice for people with severe RA that does not respond to NSAIDs. It often leads to improvement within a month—much more quickly than antimalarials, gold, or penicillamine (see page 44). The once-weekly oral dose of 7.5 to 20 mg usually is well tolerated.

The most common side effects of methotrexate are irritation of the stomach and inflammation of the mucous membranes of the mouth. Rarely, the drug produces an extremely dangerous toxic reaction that may include lung inflammation, bone marrow suppression, and severe liver damage.

Because methotrexate may harm the liver, a biopsy—removal of a tiny sample of the liver to check for damage—was previously recommended every two to three years for people taking this drug. A number of studies now suggest that regular liver biopsies (which are expensive and can cause complications of their own) are unnecessary. The studies found that even if a biopsy were performed every five years, the risk of biopsy complications was equal to the chance of finding liver damage. Instead, experts recommend periodic blood tests to monitor liver function. A biopsy is performed only if blood tests indicate liver damage. Doctors also may take a baseline chest x-ray for comparison purposes should lung complications develop from the drug, especially if the patient has underlying lung disease.

Despite some concern that methotrexate might increase the risk of such blood cancers as leukemia or lymphoma, this association appears unlikely, according to a recent study. If any link does exist, the authors of the study state that it would be small and unrelated to the dosage or length of methotrexate therapy.

Based on recent studies, low-dose folic acid supplements are recommended as an inexpensive way to reduce methotrexate side effects. The supplements appear to reduce the liver toxicity of the drug. Because high doses of folic acid can mask the warning symptoms of vitamin B_{12} deficiency, people should not start taking these supplements without first checking with their doctor.

Research on the use of methotrexate to treat RA may in fact result in a major change in the approach rheumatologists take in starting drug therapy. An analysis of results from 11 clinical trials indicates that, contrary to current practice, RA should be treated aggressively in the initial stages of the disease. The analysis found that methotrexate produced major improvements in 44% of patients during the first year of the disease, in 51% of those who had the disease for one to two years, and in 42% of those who had the disease for two to five years. The beneficial effect dropped dramatically after five years; just 29% of people who had RA for more than five years were helped by methotrexate. Among people taking a placebo, improvements were seen in less than 6% of those who had RA for five years or more. If these findings are borne out by further research, potent drugs may be prescribed early in the course of the disease to gain better control of symptoms. Additional studies have shown that methotrexate is more effective when combined with other drugs, such as cyclosporine, leflunomide (Arava), etanercept (Enbrel), infliximab (Remicade), or adalimumab (Humira).

NEW RESEARCH

Rheumatoid Arthritis Raises Risk of Heart Attacks

Women who have rheumatoid arthritis (RA) have about twice the risk of heart attacks as women without RA, but they have no increased risk of strokes, according to new research.

The research, which began in 1976, involved nearly 115,000 female nurses (age 30 to 55) who had never had a heart attack or stroke. Over the next 20 years, women who had RA were more than twice as likely to have a heart attack as women who did not have RA. Those with RA also were more likely to be older, have a parent with a history of a heart attack before age 60, exercise less, be current or past smokers, not drink, and have used hormone replacement therapy, all factors that can increase the risk of heart attacks. But even after adjusting for these factors, women with RA still had a twofold greater risk of heart attacks.

The inflammation experienced by people with RA may also contribute to the inflammatory process involved in atherosclerosis, the buildup of deposits in artery walls that can lead to heart attacks.

Because of their increased risk of heart disease, people with RA may need to take an aggressive approach to controlling other heart disease risk factors, like elevated blood cholesterol levels, high blood pressure, and smoking.

CIRCULATION
Volume 107, page 1303
March 11, 2003

Minocycline. Minocycline is a tetracycline antibiotic that has been studied for use in RA. It is unclear how it might work but is believed to reduce inflammation. Some (but not all) studies have shown a reduction in symptoms with minocycline, and one study suggested that the medication has the ability to slow joint damage. Further research is needed to determine the exact role of minocycline in the treatment of RA.

Penicillamine. Penicillamine (Cuprimine, Depen) has proven effective—particularly in studies carried out in the United Kingdom—in people who are unresponsive to all other measures. Its use is limited, however, by adverse reactions that occur in about half the people taking this drug. Side effects include fever, rash, mouth ulcers, loss of taste, protein in the urine, and low blood levels of white blood cells and platelets. The usual dosage is 125 to 1,500 mg/day.

Sulfasalazine. Sulfasalazine (Azulfidine EN-tabs) appears to suppress the immune system response that is activated in RA and also acts as an anti-inflammatory agent. The usual dosage of sulfasalazine is 1.5 to 4 g per day; the drug generally does not take effect for at least four weeks. The dosage may be raised after 12 weeks if patients still do not feel better. Because of adverse effects—which include skin rash, headache, nausea, vomiting, stomach problems, loss of appetite, and decreased sperm count—patients should be monitored closely for the first three months of therapy. Less frequent side effects include itching, fever, anemia, and skin eruptions and discoloration. Based on x-rays of joints, clinical trials have shown sulfasalazine to be as effective as gold salts.

New Drug Treatments

Etanercept (Enbrel), leflunomide (Arava), anakinra (Kineret), and adalimumab (Humira) are drugs that not only treat the symptoms of RA but also have been shown to slow the associated structural damage in the joint that occurs over time.

Etanercept, anakinra, and adalimumab must be injected (leflunomide comes in pill form). At first, a health care professional should administer the injections. Only with a physician's approval and after instruction by a health care professional should people self-inject the medication. The drug is injected into the layer of fat directly under the skin, and the site of the injection should be rotated regularly. (Common injection sites include the upper arm, thigh, and abdomen.) The drugs must be refrigerated but should not be frozen.

Infliximab (Remicade), another new medication for RA, originally

Recommended Tests for People Taking Medication for Rheumatoid Arthritis

Treatment of rheumatoid arthritis (RA) often involves the use of nonsteroidal anti-inflammatory drugs (NSAIDs), disease-modifying antirheumatic drugs (DMARDs), and corticosteroids to relieve pain, reduce inflammation, and slow progression of joint damage. But these medications can be toxic to the liver, kidneys, and bone marrow. Periodic blood and urine tests can usually detect toxicity before permanent damage occurs. This table summarizes the tests you should have—and how often you should undergo them—when you are receiving drug treatment for RA.

Medication	Recommended Test(s)	How Often Performed
adalimumab (Humira)	None	Not applicable
anakinra (Kineret)	Blood test: CBC	Once a month for the first 3 months; then every 3 months for up to 1 year
auranofin (Ridaura)	Blood test: CBC Urine test: protein	Every 4 to 12 weeks
azathioprine (Imuran)	Blood test: CBC	Every 1 to 2 weeks after changes in dosage; otherwise, every 1 to 3 months
corticosteroids such as prednisone (Deltasone, Prednisone Intensol, Sterapred)	Urine test: glucose	Once a year
cyclosporine (Neoral, Sandimmune)	Blood test: creatinine Blood tests: CBC, liver function, and potassium	Every 2 weeks until a stable dosage is reached; once a month thereafter Periodically
etanercept (Enbrel)	None	Not applicable
gold sodium thiomalate (Myochrysine)	Blood test: CBC Urine test: protein	Every 1 to 2 weeks for the first 20 weeks; then at the time of each (or every other) injection
hydroxychloroquine (Plaquenil)	Eye exam	At least once a year
infliximab (Remicade)	None	Not applicable
leflunomide (Arava)	Blood tests: CBC, creatinine, and liver function	Once a month for the first 6 months; every 1 to 2 months thereafter
methotrexate (Rheumatrex)	Blood tests: CBC, creatinine, and liver function	Once a month for the first 6 months; every 1 to 2 months thereafter
minocycline (Minocin)	None	Not applicable
NSAIDs, including aspirin and COX-2 inhibitors	Blood test: CBC Blood test: liver function*	Once a year Within the first 8 weeks; periodically thereafter
penicillamine (Cuprimine, Depen)	Blood test: CBC Urine test: protein	Every 2 weeks until a stable dosage is reached; every 1 to 3 months thereafter
Prosorba column	Blood test: CBC	Periodically
sulfasalazine (Azulfidine EN-tabs)	Blood test: CBC	Every 2 to 4 weeks for the first 3 months; every 3 months thereafter

CBC = complete blood cell count. Includes hematocrit, hemoglobin, and number of white blood cells (including differential), red blood cells, and platelets; COX-2 = cyclooxygenase-2.
* Required only for diclofenac (Voltaren).

Source: *Arthritis & Rheumatism,* February 2002, pp. 334–335.

was approved for the treatment of Crohn's disease, a disorder of the gastrointestinal tract. While this medication can treat the symptoms of RA, it is not known to slow the progression of the disease. The drug must be administered intravenously by a doctor or nurse.

Etanercept. Etanercept inhibits the action of a protein called tumor necrosis factor, which invades the joints of people with RA. In one six-month clinical trial of 234 people, 62% of people taking etanercept experienced at least a 20% reduction in symptoms such as pain and joint swelling compared with 23% of those taking a placebo. Injections of 25-mg doses are administered twice weekly, about three to four days apart. Patients may start to see results two weeks to three months after treatment begins.

Etanercept should be used with caution in people with heart failure because the drug has the potential to worsen their condition. The drug can also cause allergic reactions such as hives. Because serious infections have been reported in people using etanercept, it might not be an appropriate treatment for people who are susceptible to infection because of a weakened immune system. Serious neurological problems, including multiple sclerosis and aplastic anemia (anemia caused by reduced production of red blood cells by the bone marrow), have also been reported. People taking the drug also need to be monitored by a doctor for neurological symptoms such as confusion, numbness, changes in vision, and difficulty walking. These symptoms may be signs of a rare but serious side effect called demyelination, in which the fatty sheath that coats nerve fibers begins to disintegrate. Common side effects are injection site reactions and headache.

Leflunomide. The drug leflunomide, which blocks an inflammation-causing enzyme, is taken orally once a day. Patients start a leflunomide regimen with 100 mg a day for three days before going on maintenance therapy of 10 to 20 mg per day. The drug often begins to work within four weeks but may take more than eight weeks in some people.

In a clinical trial of 482 people with RA, more than 40% experienced at least a 20% reduction in their symptoms. The most common side effects reported were diarrhea, loss or thinning of hair, and rash. Leflunomide can also elevate liver enzymes (a sign of liver function problems), and people with liver disease should not take the drug. People taking leflunomide should have regular liver tests.

Furthermore, the drug should not be used by women who are pregnant or could become pregnant and are not using reliable contraception, because it may cause birth defects or fetal death. People prone to infection are not good candidates for leflunomide.

In a year-long study of 402 people, investigators found that leflunomide was as effective as methotrexate in treating the symptoms of RA; both had about a 50% success rate compared with 26% for placebo. However, the side effects of the two drugs are different, and people who do not tolerate one drug may benefit from the other.

Anakinra. Anakinra blocks the activity of a protein called interleukin-1. This protein is produced in excess amounts in people with RA and contributes to the pain, inflammation, and joint damage associated with the disease. The drug, which requires daily injections, is recommended only for adults who have not experienced symptom relief with at least one other DMARD, such as methotrexate, etanercept, or infliximab.

The effectiveness of anakinra has been evaluated in three randomized, placebo-controlled trials involving nearly 1,400 people (age 18 and older) with active RA. In these studies, a 20% improvement in symptoms after six months was seen in 34% to 43% of people taking anakinra (either alone or in combination with methotrexate) and 22% to 27% of those taking a placebo. On average, symptom relief with anakinra occurred within three months of beginning the treatment.

The most common side effects of anakinra in the clinical trials were redness, bruising, inflammation, and pain at the site of injection. These effects, which occurred in about 70% of patients, were mild and lasted for two to four weeks.

Anakinra also increased the risk of infection. Serious infections, such as pneumonia, occurred in about 2% of patients on anakinra, compared with less than 1% of those on a placebo. To reduce infection risk, anakinra should not be used while taking etanercept or infliximab—two DMARDs that also increase susceptibility to infection. In addition, anakinra should not be started in people with an active infection or continued if a serious infection develops (for example, one that requires treatment with an antibiotic).

In a small percentage of patients, anakinra can cause neutropenia (a decrease in infection-fighting white blood cells called neutrophils). To monitor for this side effect, your doctor should test your blood before beginning treatment with anakinra; after treatment is begun, tests should be done monthly for the first three months and then every three months for up to a year.

Anakinra is taken by injection once a day at a dosage of 100 mg. As with etanercept, a health professional will instruct you or your

---

NEW RESEARCH

Rheumatoid Arthritis Increases Mortality Risk

People with rheumatoid arthritis (RA) are at greater risk for dying of any cause than those with osteoarthritis (OA) or without arthritis, according to a new study. RA patients were also more likely to experience cardiovascular events such as heart attacks and strokes.

When researchers examined the medical records of more than 2 million patients age 40 and older in Great Britain, they identified 3,150 men and 8,123 women with RA. Over a five-year period, people with RA were 60% to 70% more likely to die and 30% to 60% more likely to experience cardiovascular events than people with OA or people without arthritis. Previous studies have also found elevated risks for cardiovascular events and death in RA patients.

The reason for the increased risk of cardiovascular events and death in people with RA is not well understood. Possible explanations include side effects from drugs used to treat RA and chronic inflammation associated with the disease.

Based on the results of this and other studies, people with RA need to be especially vigilant about controlling any risk factors they may have for cardiovascular disease. These risk factors include elevated cholesterol levels, high blood pressure, and smoking.

THE JOURNAL OF RHEUMATOLOGY
Volume 30, page 1196
June 2003

caregiver on how to inject anakinra. If you have dexterity problems or are afraid of needles, you can use a device called a SimpleJect Auto-Injector system.

Infliximab. Infliximab is combined with methotrexate in people who do not respond sufficiently to methotrexate alone. As with etanercept, infliximab neutralizes the activity of tumor necrosis factor, thereby reducing some RA symptoms. One 30-week study included 428 people who did not respond adequately to methotrexate. The addition of infliximab to methotrexate produced at least a 20% reduction in symptoms in more than half of the patients.

Infliximab is administered by intravenous infusions, typically in an outpatient setting. After an initial infusion, patients return for a second treatment about two weeks later. They then receive a third infusion about six weeks after the first one. Thereafter, the dosage is 3 to 10 mg every eight weeks.

A recent phase II trial of infliximab for heart failure found that people taking the drug had an increased rate of mortality and hospitalization for worsening heart failure. In response, the manufacturer notified doctors that people with heart failure should not begin using the drug and that infliximab therapy should be reevaluated for people with heart failure and some other heart conditions.

As with etanercept, people taking infliximab must be monitored by their doctor for neurological symptoms such as confusion, numbness, changes in vision, and difficulty walking. Also, as with etanercept, people taking infliximab may develop serious infections, and people who suffer from chronic infections or take immunosuppressive therapy should consider other RA therapies. Because infliximab can cause latent tuberculosis to develop into full-blown tuberculosis, patients should receive a tuberculin skin test before beginning therapy. Other reported side effects with infliximab include headache and acute reactions to the infusion.

Adalimumab. Like etanercept and infliximab, adalimumab works by blocking tumor necrosis factor. It is used in people who have not responded adequately to other medications, such as methotrexate. It can be used alone, or in combination with methotrexate or other DMARDs.

In one six-month study of 544 people, 46% of people taking adalimumab experienced at least a 20% reduction of symptoms, compared with 19% taking a placebo. In a twelve-month study of 619 people, a combination of methotrexate and adalimumab produced a response rate of 59%, compared with 24% for placebo plus methotrexate.

A 40-mg dose of the drug is injected once every other week. Common side effects are irritation at the injection site, sinus infections, headache, and nausea. Like etanercept and infliximab, adalimumab may produce rare side effects such as serious infections (including tuberculosis), nervous system diseases, cancer, lupus-like symptoms, and allergic reactions.

Prosorba Column

The Prosorba column, which has been available since 1999, is a treatment option for people with RA that does not respond to medication. Similar to kidney dialysis, this unusual type of therapy removes from the blood immune proteins that are believed to cause inflammation. The whole procedure takes approximately two hours and must be performed once a week for 12 weeks to be effective. No clinical studies have yet proven the long-term effectiveness or safety of the Prosorba column.

Surgery

People with RA can benefit from the same surgical procedures used to treat OA (see pages 19–26). Two additional options for people with RA are synovectomy and resection.

Synovectomy. This procedure—performed mostly in people whose RA has not responded to medication—involves the removal of the inflamed synovial membrane in the elbow, shoulder, hip, or knee. Synovectomy prevents the joint stiffness and destruction of cartilage, ligaments, tendons, and bone caused by substances released from the diseased synovial cells. Synovectomy is not as complicated a procedure as joint replacement; it is not considered a permanent cure because the synovial membrane can grow back within several years. The procedure can be performed through either a standard incision (open surgery) or several smaller incisions using special instruments (arthroscopy), depending on the size of the joint. Medication is still required after synovectomy to reduce the chance that synovitis will recur.

Resection. In this procedure, all or part of a bone is removed from a joint in the hand, wrist, elbow, toe, or ankle. Resection is most commonly performed to relieve pain in people with RA. Recovery times vary but may be as long as several weeks.

Alternative and Complementary Treatments

People with RA often turn to therapies that are outside the medical mainstream, especially when conventional medications offer

NEW RESEARCH

Rheumatologists and Hand Surgeons Differ in Their Approach

Rheumatologists and hand surgeons often disagree on when to perform common surgical procedures for rheumatoid arthritis (RA) of the hand, according to a new study. Making the situation more confusing for patients is that when these specialists disagree, they often fail to adequately communicate their views to each other.

The clashing opinions emerged from a questionnaire sent to 280 hand surgeons and 234 rheumatologists. The two groups disagreed on when to perform procedures such as finger joint replacement, removal of the synovial lining in the finger joints, and resection of a bone in the wrist.

Nearly 75% of the rheumatologists said that hand surgeons had a "poor" understanding of medical options for RA hand deformities, and a similar percentage of hand surgeons said that rheumatologists' understanding of surgical options was inadequate. While 81% of hand surgeons said they communicated the options and plans for their patients with RA to rheumatologists, only 46% of the rheumatologists agreed with that assessment. The discrepancy was similar when the question was reversed.

The study authors called for efforts to increase communication between surgeons and rheumatologists and urged patients with RA to ask their physicians about all possible treatment options.

THE JOURNAL OF RHEUMATOLOGY
Volume 30, page 1464
July 2003

What You Can Do About Lupus

There is no cure, but proper treatment can ease symptoms and reduce complications.

The word "lupus" usually refers to a specific type of lupus called systemic lupus erythematosus (SLE). However, there are other types of lupus, including discoid lupus (which produces disk-like lesions on the skin, but the rest of the body is unaffected), drug-induced lupus (a condition similar to SLE, but the symptoms fade when the patient stops taking the offending drug), and neonatal lupus (a rare condition affecting the newborns of some women with immune system diseases).

All forms of lupus are autoimmune diseases—conditions in which immune cells attack a person's own tissues. The varied symptoms of SLE—which can include joint pain and disorders of the skin, kidneys, blood, lungs, and nervous system—typically begin between the ages of 15 and 44, but about 15% of cases begin at age 55 or older. About 90% of people with SLE are women, and the condition is about two to three times more common in blacks, Hispanics, Native Americans, and Asians than in whites. An estimated 1.4 million people in the United States have some form of lupus; roughly 1 in 250 to 1,000 adults has SLE.

The cause of SLE is unknown, but experts suspect that it results from complex interactions among environmental, genetic, and hormonal factors. While there is no cure for SLE, it can often be managed effectively, and 80% to 90% of people with the disease have a normal life span.

Symptoms

In SLE, immune cells attack tissues in different parts of the body, causing inflammation, injury, and pain. For many patients, only one or a limited number of body parts is affected. Almost all SLE patients experience joint soreness (arthralgia) or joint inflammation (arthritis). The arthritis—which typically occurs in the hands, wrists, or knees—can sometimes cause joint deformity.

About 90% of patients also have skin problems, such as disk-like lesions or a butterfly rash across the face. A similar percentage experiences fatigue or fever. Half of SLE patients develop persistent kidney inflammation (lupus nephritis), which may result in kidney failure that requires dialysis or a kidney transplant.

The lining of the lungs, heart, or abdominal cavity may also become inflamed. Sometimes, anxiety, depression, seizures, or psychosis may result from the effects of SLE on the nervous system.

As many as 40% of people with SLE may develop accelerated or premature atherosclerosis, a narrowing of the arteries with plaque. Many patients also have blood disorders, such as low levels of platelets, red blood cells, or white blood cells. In addition, people with SLE produce an antibody that can promote blood clot formation, raising the risk of heart attack and stroke. Another potential consequence of SLE is osteoporosis, which increases the risk of bone fractures, especially in people who take the corticosteroid medication prednisone (Deltasone and other brands).

People with SLE do not experience their symptoms continuously; periodic flare-ups are followed by periods of symptom remission. Some 20% to 30% of SLE patients experience only bouts of mild symptoms that affect the skin or joints. However, in 50% to 75% of cases, the disorder affects a major organ, such as the kidneys,

insufficient relief of symptoms or cause troubling side effects.

The problem is that few of these nontraditional treatments have been evaluated in well-designed clinical trials. For this reason, the American College of Rheumatology (ACR) does not recommend any complementary or alternative treatments for RA.

The ACR's recommendation, however, may change with time. Numerous trials of complementary therapies are being conducted, some with funding from the U.S. government's National Institutes of Health through the National Center for Complementary and Alternative Medicine. If these trials produce compelling evidence of the benefits of a treatment that is now considered nontraditional, the treatment could become part of standard therapy.

lungs, or heart. Factors that may exacerbate flare-ups include certain medications, sunlight, infections, and hormonal changes that occur with menstruation or pregnancy.

Diagnosis
To diagnose SLE, your doctor will ask about your medical history, perform a physical examination, and order laboratory tests. Laboratory tests may include a complete blood count, blood chemistries, blood tests for certain antibodies, and urinalysis. SLE patients commonly have evidence of antinuclear antibodies—proteins that attack the cell nuclei—in their blood. Because some healthy people test positive for antinuclear antibodies, doctors typically test for other antibodies that are more specific for SLE. But not everyone with SLE will test positive for these more specific antibodies. Biopsies of the skin or kidneys may also be required.

No single symptom or test is indicative of SLE. In order to make a diagnosis, a patient must have at least 4 of the following 11 criteria: 1) malar rash (butterfly rash across the cheeks and nose), 2) discoid rash (disk-like scars, typically on sun-exposed areas), 3) skin that is sensitive to light, 4) ulcers in the mouth,

5) arthritis, 6) serositis (inflammation of the lining of the lungs, heart, or abdominal cavity), 7) kidney disorder, 8) neurological disorder, 9) blood disorder, 10) immunological disorder (positive test for certain antibodies), and 11) a positive antinuclear antibody test.

Treatment
Lifestyle measures to improve symptoms of SLE include regular use of a high SPF sunscreen, avoiding excess sun exposure, getting sufficient rest (8 to 10 hours of sleep per day), spacing out strenuous activities to avoid fatigue, exercising, and eating a healthy diet. However, medications are almost always needed to help prevent or control flare-ups. Medications may also be required to prevent heart disease.

For mild symptoms, such as joint or muscle pain, aspirin or other non-steroidal anti-inflammatory drugs (NSAIDs) may be all that is needed. Often, however, treatment for SLE involves a combination of medications including the following:
- oral, topical, injected, or intravenous corticosteroids to suppress inflammation and the immune system;
- immunosuppressive drugs such as azathioprine (Imuran) and cyclophosphamide (Cytoxan and

Neosar) to suppress the immune system and manage flare-ups; and
- antimalarial drugs such as hydroxychloroquine (Plaquenil) to address joint and skin problems and other symptoms.

However, each of these drugs has potentially dangerous side effects. The risk of these side effects is increased when the drugs are used at high doses for extended periods. Therefore, these medications are typically prescribed at the lowest effective dose for the shortest possible time.

Doctors must individualize treatment for each patient to balance the need for relieving symptoms and preventing flare-ups with the risk of long-term side effects. These side effects can include liver or kidney problems with NSAIDs; osteoporosis, high blood pressure, high blood sugar, and infections with corticosteroids; increased risk of infection and cancer with immunosuppressive drugs; and retinal damage with antimalarials. The many patients with SLE who must take these drugs for years need to work closely with their doctors, even during times of symptom remission, to ensure they are keeping in check the long-term complications of both the disease and its treatments.

In the meantime, people who wish to try complementary therapies should do so with caution. They should be sure to tell their doctor about any complementary therapies they are using or plan to use and should not discontinue their regular medication without discussing it with their doctor. They also should keep an eye on the bottom line: People with arthritis spend an estimated $1 billion each year on unproven remedies.

Supplements. People should be skeptical about nutritional supplements that purport to be safe and effective treatments for arthritis. Most of them don't work, and some are dangerous, either on their own or when combined with conventional medications. Also, because supplements are not regulated by the FDA, these products might be contaminated with toxic materials or contain less than (or none of) the listed amount of the active ingredients. Some "miracle" formulas for arthritis contain corticosteroids, which is hazardous because people taking corticosteroids need to be monitored by their doctor for serious side effects.

The Arthritis Foundation warns against using arnica (*Arnica montana*); aconite (*Aconitum napellus*); adrenal, spleen, and thymus extracts; autumn crocus (*Colchicum autumnale*); 5-HTP (5-hydroxytryptophan); GHB (gamma-hydroxybutyrate); GBL (gamma-butyrolactone); L-tryptophan; chaparral; and kombucha tea. Also dangerous are megadoses of vitamins such as A and D, which become toxic at very high doses. However, this is by no means an exhaustive list of unsafe supplements.

Chondroitin sulfate and glucosamine are two supplements that have shown promising results in people with osteoarthritis (OA). However, there is no evidence for their use in treating RA.

Supplements of gamma linolenic acid (GLA) and fish oil for RA have produced slightly more encouraging results, although the few studies conducted have included only a small number of participants. The usual dosage of GLA, which is found in borage oil, evening primrose oil, and black currant oil, is about 1,800 mg a day. The active ingredients in fish oil are the omega-3 fatty acids eicosapentaenoic acid (EPA) and docosahexaenoic acid (DHA); the usual daily dosage is 3 g.

Both GLA and fish oil may cause bleeding in people who are taking warfarin (Coumadin) or NSAIDs. Evening primrose oil can lead to gastrointestinal symptoms such as indigestion, nausea, diarrhea, and abdominal pain. Fish oil can cause indigestion, bad breath, and nosebleeds; nausea and diarrhea can occur at high doses.

As mentioned above, contamination and nonstandardization are potential problems in products that are not regulated by the FDA. For example, the fish used to manufacture fish oil supplements may be contaminated with mercury, dioxin, or polychlorinated biphenyls (PCBs). Fish oils also have a tendency to become rancid, which makes the oil foul smelling and, possibly, less effective. In addition, a recent review of 20 brands of fish oil supplements by ConsumerLab, an independent testing laboratory, found that only 14 contained the amount of omega-3 fatty acids stated on the label. Likewise, GLA supplements may contain little or no GLA. You can reduce these risks by buying supplements that meet U.S. Pharmacopeia standards (look for the "USP" symbol) or by checking results from ConsumerLab at www.consumerlab.com.

Mind-body therapies. Mind-body therapies such as biofeedback, meditation, and relaxation exercises generally are safe and may temporarily reduce pain by promoting relaxation. None of these therapies has been shown to have lasting effects on arthritis, however. Likewise, massage can be relaxing and feel good on sore muscles but has only temporary effects. If you do get a massage, make sure that the massage therapist is trained and licensed, knows that you have arthritis, and avoids pressure on damaged or inflamed joints.

Acupuncture. Acupuncture, in which fine needles are inserted into specific places in the body, appears to hold some promise as a treatment for OA. However, studies on acupuncture for RA have been disappointing.

Homeopathy. In homeopathy, an agent such as poison ivy or bee venom is greatly diluted and then administered as a remedy. A randomized, controlled trial of homeopathy found that it is no more effective than a placebo for treating RA.

Treating Depression

While the pain and disability associated with arthritis can trigger depression, evidence also indicates that arthritis pain is worse when accompanied by symptoms of depression. Therefore, treating depression can have far-reaching effects for people with arthritis. Treatment options for depression include medication, psychotherapy, and exercise. Becoming more educated about one's condition also seems to reduce or prevent depression. In a study of 202 older people with arthritis, those who attended a 10-week class about the symptoms, course, and treatment of arthritis had fewer depressive symptoms at the end of the class than those in the control group.

Gout

Gout is a metabolic disease characterized by increased blood levels of uric acid, which cause recurrent bouts of acute "gouty" arthritis. The condition affects about 2.1 million Americans. In its early stages, gout usually involves a single joint; later on, a chronic arthritis can affect many joints and cause joint deformity. Gout occurs much more frequently in men, most often after age 30. In women, attacks of gout usually do not begin until after menopause. Obesity increases the risk of developing gout; about half of those with gout are 15% or more above their ideal weight.

NEW RESEARCH

Computer Use Does Not Increase Carpal Tunnel Risk

Using a computer does not appear to increase the risk of developing carpal tunnel syndrome, a new study finds. However, frequent use of the mouse may be associated with this condition, in which compression of the median nerve in the wrist causes tingling and pain.

In the largest study of computers and carpal tunnel syndrome so far, researchers surveyed more than 5,600 members of a Danish trade union whose jobs required them to use computers. At the beginning of the study, 4.8% of the participants reported tingling or numbness in the medial nerve. One year later, 5.5% reported new or worsened symptoms, but only 1.2% of the participants had symptoms in the median nerve—a rate comparable to that in the general population.

The researchers did find, however, that using the mouse 20 to 25 hours per week more than doubled the risk of carpal tunnel syndrome, and using it 25 to 30 hours per week more than tripled the risk.

The researchers say that the motion involved in computer use (repetition with no force) is the type least likely to cause carpal tunnel syndrome. However, computer use may be associated with other problems, such as wrist tendinitis or shoulder pain.

JOURNAL OF THE AMERICAN MEDICAL ASSOCIATION
Volume 289, page 2963
June 11, 2003

CAUSES OF GOUT

Gout can be divided into two types: primary and secondary. In the inherited form, known as primary gout, elevated blood levels of uric acid result from an increased production of uric acid, a reduced excretion of uric acid in the urine, or some combination of the two. In secondary gout, blood levels of uric acid are raised by use of diuretics, chronic kidney failure, or a massive release of the chemical precursors to uric acid during the rapid destruction of cells. Cell destruction of this sort may occur during cancer chemotherapy or in association with such diseases as multiple myeloma, leukemia, or psoriasis.

Acute gouty arthritis is initiated by the deposition of sodium urate crystals into a joint and its synovial membrane. White blood cells (specifically, polymorphonuclear cells) enter the joint, engulf the urate crystals, and release a number of substances that trigger inflammation and an acute attack of arthritis. Urate crystals can also accumulate in many other sites, such as the kidneys, tendons, bones, and directly beneath the skin. Accumulations of urate create characteristic lesions called tophi—uric acid crystals surrounded by cells that amass to defend against the deposited "foreign body." Chronic gouty arthritis results when a joint is damaged by the formation of tophi within and around the joint. If gout is chronic, osteoarthritis often develops in the joint.

A high blood level of uric acid (hyperuricemia) is a consistent finding in people with gout, but many people with persistent hyperuricemia never develop gout. In addition, it appears that a rapid drop—as well as a rapid rise—in blood uric acid levels can precipitate an attack of acute gout.

Uric acid kidney stones often result from the excessive excretion of uric acid in the urine, and deposition of urates in the kidneys can eventually lead to kidney damage and failure.

Pseudogout

Pseudogout is caused by acute inflammation due to the accumulation of crystals of calcium pyrophosphate (rather than uric acid) within a joint. (Blood uric acid levels are usually normal in individuals with pseudogout.) The disorder is often first suspected from x-rays that show calcification of the cartilage (chondrocalcinosis). Diagnosis is confirmed when microscopic examination of fluid taken from the affected joint reveals the typical calcium pyrophosphate crystals.

The disorder can lead to recurrent attacks of acute arthritis, generally involving large joints such as the knee and wrist. It occurs most often in people over age 60, and symptoms are limited to the joints. Pseudogout is frequently associated with an underlying metabolic abnormality, such as diabetes, an underactive thyroid, an overactive parathyroid, excessive tissue deposits of iron (hemochromatosis) or copper (Wilson's disease), and true gout.

No known medication can prevent pseudogout by stopping the formation of joint crystals. Treatment is limited to easing the pain with aspirin or other NSAIDs. When swelling and pain persist, removal of fluid from the joint and steroid injection may provide relief.

SYMPTOMS OF GOUT

Acute attacks of gout usually occur without warning, often at night. Gouty arthritis of the big toe (podagra) is particularly common; the big toe is affected at some time in 75% of people with gout. Acute arthritis also can affect the knee, ankle, and foot; several joints may be involved simultaneously. Progressively severe joint pain is accompanied by swelling, extreme tenderness, warmth and redness of the skin overlying the joint, and moderate fever. Relief is obtained quickly with drugs. If left untreated, however, an acute attack can last for days.

Each attack may be followed by months or years in which the person is free from further episodes, but these pain-free intervals tend to become shorter over time. Progress of the disease is particularly rapid when gout begins before age 50. Unless treated, gout often progresses to its chronic stage, which is characterized by loss of function and deformity of joints. People with gout also have an increased incidence of high blood pressure, kidney disease, diabetes, and atherosclerosis (a buildup of plaque in the arteries that can lead to a heart attack or stroke). Between 10% and 20% of people with gouty arthritis have uric acid kidney stones.

DIAGNOSIS OF GOUT

A diagnosis of gout is strongly suspected from the typical symptoms and appearance of an affected joint. After people have suffered several attacks of gouty arthritis, a physical exam may reveal tophi in the earlobe, knee, foot, or elbow. Blood tests show an increased level of uric acid and, during an acute attack, an elevated sedimentation rate ("sed" rate) and white blood cell count. The diagnosis is confirmed by the presence of urate crystals in a microscopic examination

NEW RESEARCH

Cigarette Smoking Aggravates Lupus

People with systemic lupus erythematosus (SLE) who smoke have another reason to quit: New research shows that tobacco significantly increases the severity of the disease. Previous studies have strongly linked smoking with the development of SLE.

In this study, researchers interviewed 111 people with SLE—35 current smokers, 36 former smokers, and 40 people who never smoked—to determine the severity of their symptoms. They also assessed the amount of damage the disease had caused to major organ systems. All the participants were age 40 or older, and 95% were women.

Disease activity scores were more than 60% higher for current smokers than for former smokers and people who never smoked. The smokers also appeared to have more organ damage than those in the other two groups, although this difference was not statistically significant.

The researchers said they weren't surprised that smoking exacerbates SLE, since cigarette smoke contains many toxic chemicals that damage cells. They strongly advise patients with SLE to avoid all tobacco products.

THE JOURNAL OF RHEUMATOLOGY
Volume 30, page 1215
June 2003

Drugs for the Treatment of Gout 2004

Drug Type	Generic Name	Brand Name	Average Daily Dosage*	Wholesale Cost (Generic Cost)†
Antigout	colchicine	Available only as a generic	**Prevention of an attack** *Oral:* 0.6 to 1.2 mg *Injection:* 0.5 to 2 mg **Treatment of an attack** *Oral:* 0.5 to 1.2 mg for the first dose; then 0.5 to 0.6 mg every one or two hours until side effects develop or a maximum dosage of 6 mg is reached *Injection:* 1 to 2 mg for the first dose; then 0.5 to 1 mg every 6 to 12 hours to a maximum of 4 mg	(0.6 mg: $22)
Combination Drug	probenecid/ colchicine	Available only as a generic	*Oral:* 1 or 4 tablets	(500 mg/0.5 mg: $84)
Corticosteroids‡	prednisone	Deltasone Prednicot Prednisone Intensol Concentrate Sterapred Sterapred DS	*Oral:* 20 to 30 mg for 7 to 10 days	10 mg: $7 ($10) 10 mg: $4 ($10) 5 mg/mL, 30 mL: $31 5 mg: $43 10 mg: $49 ($10)
	triamcinolone	Aristospan IA Kenalog-10 Kenalog-40	*Injection:* 10 to 40 mg per joint	20 mg/mL, 5 mL: $21 10 mg/mL, 5 mL: $8 40 mg/mL, 5 mL: $33

How the Drug Works	Special Instructions	Possible Side Effects
Prevents or relieves the inflammation that results from the accumulation of uric acid crystals in a joint.	To prevent or treat acute attacks of gout. Used for treatment when NSAIDs and corticosteroids are ineffective or cannot be tolerated. Most effective when taken within the first 12 hours of an acute attack. Should not be used by people who have kidney or liver disease or are heavy drinkers. To prevent serious side effects, do not take larger doses or use more often than directed by your doctor. **For prevention:** Should be taken with a xanthine oxidase inhibitor or a uricosuric drug (see pages 55–60) to prevent the buildup of tophi. **For treatment:** Stop taking the medication once pain is relieved. Also stop the medication if diarrhea, vomiting, nausea, or stomach pain occurs or if the maximum dosage is reached before pain is relieved. Do not resume taking colchicine for prevention of gout for at least three days after taking the drug orally and at least seven days after an injection.	Common side effects include diarrhea, nausea, vomiting, and stomach pain. Check with your doctor if these side effects last more than three hours after stopping the medication. Contact your doctor immediately if you develop black, tarry stools; blood in urine or stools; difficulty breathing when exercising; fever with or without chills; headache; large hive-like swellings on the face, eyelids, mouth, lips, or tongue; pinpoint red spots on skin; sores, ulcers, or white spots on lips or in mouth; sore throat; unusual bleeding or bruising; or unusual tiredness or weakness.
Probenecid lowers blood levels of uric acid by increasing the excretion of uric acid by the kidneys, while colchicine prevents the inflammation that results from the accumulation of uric acid crystals in a joint.	To prevent acute attacks of gout. Not helpful for the treatment of acute gout attacks. Should not be used by those with a history of kidney stones. Should not be started during an acute attack of gout. Do not take aspirin or drink alcoholic beverages while taking this medication, unless you have your doctor's permission. To prevent serious side effects, do not take larger doses or use more often than directed by your doctor. To decrease the risk of kidney stones and other kidney problems, drink at least 10 to 12 glasses of fluid a day. Alternatively, your doctor may prescribe a medication that makes urine less acidic. If upset stomach occurs, take the medication with food. If this doesn't help, an antacid may be used.	Common side effects include mild diarrhea, headache, loss of appetite, mild nausea or vomiting, and stomach pain. Stop taking the medication and contact your doctor if gastrointestinal side effects become severe while taking four or more tablets a day. Also contact your doctor immediately if you experience any of the following: rapid or irregular breathing; puffiness or swelling of the eyelids or around the eyes; tightness in chest or wheezing; changes in the skin color of the face; or skin rash, hives, or itching.
Decreases the formation, release, and activity of compounds (including prostaglandins) that produce inflammation in the body.	To treat acute attacks of gout. Usually prescribed when NSAIDs are ineffective or cannot be tolerated. Do not drink alcohol while taking prednisone, unless you have your doctor's permission. To prevent side effects, do not take more or less of the medication, use it more often, or take it longer than directed by your doctor. Take prednisone with food to prevent stomach upset. Following an injection of triamcinolone, be careful not to put too much stress or strain on the joint for 24 to 48 hours.	Common side effects include decreased or blurred vision, frequent urination, increased thirst, increased or greatly diminished appetite, indigestion, nervousness, and restlessness. Check with your doctor if you experience any of these effects. Contact your doctor if you notice that redness or swelling at the site of the injection persists or gets worse.

Drugs for the Treatment of Gout 2004 (continued)

Drug Type	Generic Name	Brand Name	Average Daily Dosage*	Wholesale Cost (Generic Cost)†
Nonsteroidal anti-inflammatory drugs§	indomethacin	Indocin Indocin SR	*Oral:* 100 to 150 mg *Rectal:* 50 to 200 mg	50 mg: $110 ($55) 75 mg: $237 ($193)
	naproxen	Aleve Anaprox Naprosyn	*Oral:* 825 mg *Oral:* 750 mg	220 mg: $9¶ (250 mg: $80) 275 mg: $101 ($85) 250 mg: $106 ($80)
Uricosuric drugs	probenecid	Available only as a generic	*Oral:* 500 to 3,000 mg	(500 mg: $83)
	sulfinpyrazone	Available only as a generic	*Oral:* 100 to 800 mg	(100 mg: $95)
Xanthine oxidase inhibitor	allopurinol	Zyloprim	*Oral:* 100 to 800 mg	100 mg: $29 ($24)

* These dosages represent an average range for the treatment of gout. The precise effective dosage varies from patient to patient and depends on many factors. Do not make any changes in your medication without consulting your doctor.

† Average wholesale prices to pharmacists for 100 tablets or capsules (unless otherwise indicated) of the dosage strength listed. Costs to consumers are higher. If a generic version is available, the cost is listed in parentheses. Source: *Red Book, 2003* (Medical Economics Data, publishers).

‡ Any corticosteroid can be used to treat an acute attack of gout. Two commonly used corticosteroids (one administered orally; the other by injection) are listed here. Other corticosteroids include betamethasone (Celestone, Selestoject), cortisone (Cortone), dexamethasone (Decadron and other brands), hydrocortisone (Cortef and other brands), methylprednisolone (Medrol and other brands), and prednisolone (Delta-Cortef and other brands). Consult your doctor regarding the appropriate dosage of these corticosteroids for the treatment of gout.

§ Any nonsteroidal anti-inflammatory drug (NSAID) can be used to treat an acute attack of gout. Two commonly used NSAIDs are listed here. For a list of other NSAIDs, see the chart on pages 18–19. Consult your doctor regarding the appropriate dosage of these NSAIDs for the treatment of gout.

¶ Cost of the over-the-counter version.

How The Drug Works	Special Instructions	Possible Side Effects
By interfering with the formation of prostaglandins, these drugs reduce the pain and inflammation caused by uric acid crystals in a joint.	First-choice therapy for the treatment of acute attacks of gout. To prevent side effects, do not take more of the medication, use it more often, or take it longer than directed by your doctor or the package label (if you are taking over-the-counter naproxen). To lessen stomach upset, these medications should be taken with food or an antacid (for example, Maalox). Use of these medications with alcohol may increase the risk of serious gastrointestinal side effects.	Common side effects include mild to moderate abdominal or stomach cramps, pain, or discomfort; dizziness, drowsiness, or light-headedness; mild to moderate headache; and heartburn, indigestion, nausea, or vomiting. Stop taking the medication and contact your doctor immediately if you experience one or more of the following: severe abdominal or stomach cramps, pain or burning; black, tarry stools; severe and continuing nausea, heartburn, or indigestion; vomiting of blood or material that resembles coffee grounds; or very fast or irregular breathing, gasping for breath, wheezing, or fainting. Also contact your doctor immediately if you have chills, fever, muscle aches or pains, or other flu-like symptoms, particularly if they occur shortly before or together with a skin rash.
Lower blood levels of uric acid by increasing the excretion of uric acid by the kidneys.	Used to prevent acute attacks of gout and prevent or treat other health conditions that are associated with too much uric acid in the body. Not helpful for the treatment of acute gout attacks. Should not be used by those with a history of kidney stones. Most effective in people whose urine contains small amounts of uric acid and those who have good kidney function. Should not be started during an acute attack of gout. Gout attacks may continue during the first three to six months of treatment. These attacks can be minimized by taking low doses of colchicine or NSAIDs. Do not take aspirin or drink alcoholic beverages while taking this medication unless you have your doctor's permission. To decrease the risk of kidney stones and other kidney problems, drink at least 10 to 12 glasses of fluid a day. Alternatively, your doctor may prescribe a medication that makes urine less acidic. If upset stomach occurs, take the medication with food. If this doesn't help, an antacid may be used.	Common side effects of probenecid include headache; joint pain, redness, or swelling; loss of appetite; and mild nausea or vomiting. Contact your doctor immediately if you develop any of the following while taking probenecid: rapid or irregular breathing; puffiness or swelling of the eyelids or around the eyes; shortness of breath, trouble breathing, tightness in chest, or wheezing; changes in skin color of the face; or skin rash, hives or itching. Common side effects of sulfinpyrazone include joint pain, redness, or swelling; nausea or vomiting; and stomach pain. Contact your doctor immediately if you develop any of the following while taking sulfinpyrazone: shortness of breath, trouble breathing, tightness in chest or wheezing; sores, ulcers, or white spots on lips or in mouth; sore throat and fever with or without chills; swollen or painful glands; or unusual bleeding or bruising.
Lowers blood levels of uric acid by reducing the body's production of uric acid.	Used to prevent acute attacks of gout and prevent or treat other health conditions, such as kidney stones and other kidney problems, that are associated with too much uric acid in the body. Not helpful for the treatment of acute gout attacks. Most effective in people whose urine contains large amounts of uric acid. Should not be started during an acute attack of gout. Gout attacks may continue during the first three to six months of treatment. These attacks can be minimized by taking low doses of colchicine or NSAIDs. If upset stomach occurs, take the medication after meals.	Common side effects include skin rash, skin sores, hives, and itching. Contact your doctor immediately if you develop these problems or chills, fever, joint pain, muscle aches and pains, sore throat, or nausea or vomiting at the same time as or shortly after a skin rash.

of fluid removed from an affected joint. X-rays usually appear normal at first, but later in the course of the disease the presence of tophi may produce "punched-out," or eroded, areas in bones.

PREVENTION OF GOUT ATTACKS

For acute attacks of gouty arthritis, prevention is the cornerstone of treatment. Fortunately, much is known about preventing flares. Another important goal is preventing urate kidney stones and kidney damage due to the deposition of urate in the kidneys.

Diet

Many foods contain purines, which can be converted to uric acid in the body. It was formerly thought that attacks of gout were provoked by eating large amounts of purine-rich foods, such as liver, anchovies, kidney, and sweetbreads (calf's thymus or pancreas). However, avoidance of such foods has little impact on blood uric acid levels. Currently recommended preventive measures include weight control (but not periods of fasting, which can raise uric acid levels), avoidance of excessive alcohol, and enough fluid intake to maintain a urine output of at least eight cups daily (to minimize formation of uric acid stones and deposition of urate in the kidneys).

Drugs That Cause Hyperuricemia

People predisposed to gout should avoid the following medications: hydrochlorothiazide (Esidrix, HydroDIURIL); cyclosporine (Neoral, Sandimmune; an immunosuppressant used to treat RA and prevent rejection of transplanted organs); furosemide (Lasix); and high dosages of aspirin—all of which decrease uric acid excretion by the kidneys—as well as nicotinic acid, or niacin. People who need to reduce their risk of a heart attack can safely take half an aspirin tablet or a baby aspirin daily.

Drugs To Lower Uric Acid Levels

Two types of medications can lower blood uric acid levels: uricosuric agents, such as probenecid (available only as a generic) and sulfinpyrazone (Anturane), and the xanthine oxidase inhibitor allopurinol (Zyloprim). Uricosuric agents increase excretion of uric acid by the kidneys, while allopurinol partly inhibits the enzyme xanthine oxidase, which produces uric acid in the body. Measuring the amount of uric acid in the urine helps to determine which drug will be most effective. Uricosuric drugs are chosen for people with small amounts of uric acid in the urine (indicating that excretion is insufficient); allopurinol is most useful in people whose urine contains large amounts of uric acid (indicating excessive formation of uric acid). These drugs are not helpful during acute attacks of gout. In fact, drugs to lower uric acid should never be started when someone is suffering from a flare, because they may cause further attacks. Moreover, neither class of drug should be used by people who have hyperuricemia without symptoms or who have infrequent attacks of gout.

A uricosuric drug is taken daily when there is an increase in the frequency or severity of gouty arthritis. Neither drug is effective in people with poor kidney function. About 10% of patients experience adverse gastrointestinal effects; about 5% develop a fever or rash. The greatest risk from uricosuric drugs is the development of uric acid kidney stones and kidney damage from the deposition of urate crystals in the kidneys.

By rapidly lowering uric acid in the blood and urine, daily doses of allopurinol can promote the removal of urate crystals from tophi and lessen the likelihood of uric acid kidney stones. Although used to decrease the incidence of gouty arthritis in those not responding to the uricosuric agents, allopurinol can precipitate an acute attack of gout. But such attacks can be prevented by giving colchicine for a short period before allopurinol is started. Another common adverse effect is an itchy rash that, in rare cases, may turn into a potentially fatal skin disorder. (After allopurinol is started, patients should report any new rash to their doctor.) Other potential side effects include hepatitis and inflammation of small blood vessels.

Colchicine

Colchicine (0.5 or 0.6 mg taken orally one to three times daily) reduces the frequency of attacks of acute gouty arthritis without lowering blood uric acid levels. Long-term colchicine treatment is most likely to benefit those who have frequent attacks and extremely high levels of uric acid. When colchicine is used to prevent acute attacks, a xanthine oxidase inhibitor or uricosuric drug agent should also be taken to avoid the buildup of tophi (which might not be noticed without arthritic attacks to serve as a warning sign). Colchicine may also prevent acute arthritis provoked by starting drug therapy that produces a rapid reduction in uric acid levels (see below).

The most common side effects of colchicine therapy are diarrhea, vomiting, nausea, and stomach pain. Other side effects in-

NEW RESEARCH

High Doses of Anticancer Drug Effective for People With Lupus

An investigational treatment involving high-dose cyclophosphamide, an anticancer medication, has led to significant benefits for some people with moderate to severe systemic lupus erythematosus (SLE).

In a recent report from Johns Hopkins, 14 patients with SLE who did not improve with traditional treatments were given high-dose intravenous cyclophosphamide for four days. Five of them achieved a "complete response" that lasted at least through the end of the study (about 2½ years). Three of these five required no drug treatment for SLE during this period. Six patients had a partial response to the treatment, while two had no response. One patient developed kidney failure.

The researchers theorize that high doses of cyclophosphamide destroy the malfunctioning immune cells that lead to the signs and symptoms of SLE. At the same time, the medication does not affect the body's stem cells, which help form new, normally functioning immune cells. Side effects of the treatment included temporary nausea, hair loss, and fever.

Researchers at Hopkins are currently comparing the effectiveness of high-dose cyclophosphamide with a standard treatment regimen for severe lupus in a large, randomized trial.

ARTHRITIS AND RHEUMATISM
Volume 48, page 166
January 2003

clude allergic reactions, such as rash or hives; muscle aching or weakness; and signs of anemia or immune suppression, such as fever, fatigue, and chills. While such reactions are rare, they can be life-threatening and tend to occur more frequently with high doses. Since the individual dosing plan can be complicated (depending on whether the drug is used to prevent attacks or to treat an acute attack), some people find it helpful to carry a schedule of when to take their medication.

TREATMENT OF GOUT ATTACKS

When gout attacks occur, early treatment provides rapid relief. The following measures are used to treat acute gouty arthritis.

Nonsteroidal anti-inflammatory drugs. NSAIDs have replaced colchicine as the treatment of choice for acute gout (see pages 13–18 and the chart on pages 16–17). All types appear equally effective in general, but some individuals may respond better to one or another of the various NSAIDs. Intramuscular injections of ketorolac (Toradol) may also provide relief of acute gout pain.

Colchicine. Colchicine can be effective when used early in the course of an acute gout attack. The drug is taken orally every 1 to 2 hours or by injection every 6 to 12 hours until the pain stops, a specific maximal dose is reached, or the person experiences nausea, vomiting, abdominal cramping, or diarrhea. Unfortunately, side effects occur in more than 80% of patients.

Corticosteroids. Oral corticosteroids are effective but generally are used only in people who do not tolerate NSAIDs. Pain may also be relieved by injecting steroids directly into an affected joint.

Narcotic analgesics. Although not commonly needed, codeine or meperidine can provide rapid relief of severe pain while waiting for the previously mentioned drugs to take effect.

Bed rest. Patients should remain in bed for about 24 hours after symptoms abate to lessen the likelihood of recurrence, since movement can induce inflammation and trigger another attack.

Fibromyalgia Syndrome

Fibromyalgia syndrome is thought by some to be the most common rheumatic condition aside from osteoarthritis. It accounts for perhaps 15% to 20% of visits to rheumatologists. According to one estimate, 2% of Americans, or about 3.7 million people (including many older women), may have the syndrome. (A syndrome is a set of symptoms and physical findings that together characterize a particular disorder.)

Unlike true arthritis, fibromyalgia does not affect the joints. Rather, it produces pain *(algia)* in the body's fibrous *(fibro)* ligaments and tendons and in the muscles *(my)*. People with fibromyalgia have generalized pain, achiness, and stiffness all over the body. Pain may radiate from various sites that are painful when touched ("trigger points"). The trigger points are very painful, although people with fibromyalgia may not even realize these particular areas hurt until pressure is applied to them. The other main characteristic of fibromyalgia is chronic fatigue, possibly related to disturbed sleep patterns. Sufferers often complain of waking up as tired as they were when they went to sleep and remaining fatigued throughout the day.

Fibromyalgia primarily affects women—up to 90% of people visiting a doctor with symptoms of this disorder are female—and usually first occurs between the ages of 20 and 60. Because this syndrome is poorly understood and difficult to recognize, it is not unusual for many years to elapse between symptom onset and diagnosis. Fortunately, more doctors are becoming aware of the collection of symptoms that characterize fibromyalgia.

Fibromyalgia causes no inflammation, and it does not damage the joints, connective tissue, or muscles. (This lack of inflammation sets fibromyalgia apart from rheumatoid arthritis.) While pain and fatigue may be quite severe at times, fibromyalgia is not a joint-deforming disease. The disorder cannot be cured, but the symptoms can be managed. People experience significant improvement once they are accurately diagnosed and treated.

CAUSES OF FIBROMYALGIA

The cause of fibromyalgia is not known, but there are several theories. Fibromyalgia may develop following a bout of flu or other illness or after extreme physical or emotional stress. Some researchers believe that fibromyalgia results from minor, repeated trauma to the muscles that decreases blood flow to them and causes weakness and fatigue.

Another theory is that the sleep disturbance associated with fibromyalgia is the underlying cause of the syndrome. The deepest, restorative stage of sleep—delta-wave sleep—is somehow disrupted in people with fibromyalgia. When healthy volunteers were deprived of delta-wave sleep, they developed tenderness in the trigger point areas for fibromyalgia, as well as other symptoms of the disorder.

Other researchers suggest that an abnormality in the central nervous system is responsible. One possibility is a brain malfunction in the production or metabolism of the neurotransmitter serotonin, which plays an important role in some of the fibromyalgia symptoms relating to pain, mood, and sleep. Other research has suggested that women with fibromyalgia have lower levels of somatomedin C. This substance is formed in the liver upon stimulation by growth hormone, which is secreted by the pituitary gland in greatest amounts during sleep. Low blood pressure is currently under investigation as another potential cause of the symptoms of fibromyalgia.

SYMPTOMS OF FIBROMYALGIA

Pain is the primary symptom of fibromyalgia. It usually starts in one area, such as the neck or lower back, but later spreads to other parts of the body. Most often, people with fibromyalgia complain of widespread pain and achiness, similar to the symptoms of a bad bout of the flu. Sometimes the pain is described as gnawing or burning. People often feel stiffer and achier in the morning than at other times of the day. The severity of pain may vary from day to day, but most people with fibromyalgia report that some level of pain is always present. Exercise, physical or emotional stress, poor sleep, or even bad weather may increase the intensity of pain. Numbness, tingling, and the sensation of swelling of the hands are other common complaints. Fibromyalgia is also accompanied by moderate to severe fatigue. Sufferers often feel that they do not have the energy to do the things they used to do. They may be unable to walk as far or exercise as much without becoming tired.

People with fibromyalgia also have a greater incidence of certain other symptoms. For example, some people report increased allergic-type reactions to medications and substances in the environment. These reactions are not necessarily true allergies but may be due to an overly reactive central nervous system. Also, tension headaches and migraines occur more often in people with fibromyalgia.

Depression has been linked to fibromyalgia, but it is not clear whether depression causes the syndrome or is a consequence of it. (For information about psychological counseling for people with fibromyalgia, see the feature on pages 68–69.) In addition, anxiety occurs in about half of people with fibromyalgia. About one third to one half of people with fibromyalgia also have irritable bowel syndrome, a gastrointestinal disorder of unknown cause. It is characterized by abdominal bloating and pain, as well as alternating bouts of constipation and diarrhea. In addition, restless leg syndrome (a condition marked by an unpleasant aching in the legs at bedtime, accompanied by an overpowering urge to walk around for relief) may affect three quarters of fibromyalgia patients.

DIAGNOSIS OF FIBROMYALGIA

Fibromyalgia is difficult to diagnose. Unlike rheumatoid arthritis or osteoarthritis, fibromyalgia produces no visible physical changes that can be used to identify the syndrome. X-rays, biopsies of tissue samples from tender areas, and blood tests do not reveal any characteristic abnormalities. Until recently, the lack of physical evidence had led many doctors to suspect a psychological basis for the symptoms. Despite the absence of any physical or laboratory evidence, fibromyalgia is a physical disorder. Fortunately, more doctors are becoming aware of the symptoms of fibromyalgia and are better able to diagnose the condition.

Trigger Points
In 1990, the American College of Rheumatology developed a set of criteria to diagnose fibromyalgia. Widespread pain, present for at least three months, must be located on both sides of the body, both above and below the waist. Pressure of about 9 lbs. applied to at least 11 of 18 trigger points must produce pain. To apply the same amount of pressure at each point tested, the doctor may use an instrument called a dolorimeter. In most cases, the pain is not just mild discomfort but acute pain that may cause a person to flinch or cry out.

It was once thought that pressure on areas of the body as close as 1 inch away from the trigger points would not cause pain in people with fibromyalgia and that this specificity of location would help to confirm the diagnosis. However, recent research has not supported this belief. While not part of the official criteria, reports of fatigue and, in particular, of nonrestorative sleep help confirm the diagnosis.

Laboratory Tests
Because the symptoms of fibromyalgia are similar to those of many other disorders, several tests may be done to rule these out. The doctor may perform blood tests to check for an underactive thyroid,

NEW RESEARCH

Ten Days of Antibiotics Effective for Early Lyme Disease

The best treatment regimen for early Lyme disease has been unclear. Now, a trial suggests that a 10-day course of oral antibiotics is highly effective and that extending the length of therapy to 20 days or adding an intravenous antibiotic does not increase the effectiveness of treatment.

The study included 180 people with the bull's-eye rash characteristic of early Lyme disease. People were randomly assigned to one of three antibiotic regimens: 10 or 20 days of oral doxycycline, or 10 days of oral doxycycline plus one dose of intravenous ceftriaxone.

After 30 months, the rash and symptoms had resolved completely in 90% of the 10-day doxycycline group, 84% of the 20-day doxycycline group, and 87% of the doxycycline-ceftriaxone group. One person in the 10-day doxycycline group did not respond to doxycycline; this person developed Lyme meningitis and was successfully treated with two weeks of intravenous ceftriaxone. Diarrhea was more common in the doxycycline-ceftriaxone group than the other groups.

A related editorial concluded that 10 days of doxycycline is usually enough for people with early Lyme disease, although people with later-stage disease need 14 to 28 days of oral antibiotics. Intravenous ceftriaxone is required only for people who develop neurological abnormalities.

ANNALS OF INTERNAL MEDICINE
Volume 138, pages 697 and 761
May 6, 2003

rheumatoid arthritis, lupus, Lyme disease, and polymyalgia rheumatica (a disorder that causes stiffness and aching in the neck, shoulder, and hip areas; other symptoms may include fatigue, weight loss, low grade fever, and depression). Imaging tests such as magnetic resonance imaging (MRI) may not be used initially, since they are expensive and sometimes associated with misleading results in diagnosing arthritis.

Fibromyalgia is not a disorder of exclusion, meaning that the diagnosis is not made simply by ruling out other diseases. Instead, the diagnosis must be based on the criteria described above. Fibromyalgia can, of course, coexist with other illnesses. For example, up to 10% of people with rheumatoid arthritis also have fibromyalgia. If fibromyalgia-like symptoms disappear when the other disorder is treated, the symptoms were likely caused by the other condition rather than by fibromyalgia.

People who suspect they have fibromyalgia should consult a doctor who has experience with this syndrome. Some doctors are still not familiar with the diagnostic criteria for fibromyalgia, and others may apply too little or too much pressure when examining the trigger points. A rheumatologist is usually the best type of doctor to see.

TREATMENT OF FIBROMYALGIA

Despite the lack of a definitive cause, fibromyalgia symptoms can be significantly improved with a multifaceted approach. The goals are to lessen pain and improve sleep. Much of the success of treatment lies with the patient, and many people report improvement simply because a diagnosis has been made. It is reassuring for people to know that the disorder is not deforming or life-threatening and that they are able to take control of their situation.

Exercise. Getting up and moving are key to improving fibromyalgia. A lack of activity worsens symptoms because unconditioned muscles are more sensitive to pain. Although exercising may be the last thing people with fibromyalgia want to do when they feel achy and tired, studies have shown that symptoms improve after six to eight weeks of moderate aerobic exercise.

It is important not to overdo it, however. Start slowly, with perhaps 5 to 10 minutes of brisk walking a day. Gradually increase the exercise time to 30 to 40 minutes of aerobic activity at least three times a week. People whose pain is exacerbated by the jarring movements of weight-bearing exercise (such as walking or jogging) may try swimming or riding a stationary bicycle instead.

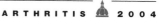

Improving sleep patterns. Many doctors recommend that people with fibromyalgia try to establish a regular sleep schedule that involves the following measures: going to bed and getting up at the same time every day; getting at least eight hours of sleep; avoiding alcohol, caffeine, and smoking in the evening; and eliminating daytime naps. This approach may not work for everyone, however, and some people may require medication. Some people have had success with low doses of tricyclic antidepressants (see pages 68–69) at bedtime; these drugs enhance the action of neurotransmitters involved in the regulation of deep sleep.

Physical therapy. In some cases, doctors may refer people with fibromyalgia to a physical therapist, either to design an exercise program or to treat particularly painful flares. Physical therapists employ several techniques. For example, in "spray and stretch," a physical therapist sprays the sore region with ethyl chloride to anesthetize it before stretching the patient's muscles.

Improving body mechanics. Many day-to-day activities and hobbies (such as needlepoint, golf, and tennis) require repetitive movements. If they are not performed correctly, they can cause fatigue and increase pain. Several sessions with a physical therapist or professional sports instructor can make sure that these activities are being done properly.

Changes to improve symptoms also can be made at the workplace. When people with fibromyalgia were surveyed to determine which job-related activities aggravated their symptoms, prolonged tasks or repetitive ones that required working under adverse conditions—such as at night or in the cold—were the most troublesome. Working on an assembly line and typing are two common causes of problems.

To help prevent a symptom flare, people with fibromyalgia should not overdo any activity. Frequently changing the types of tasks performed is a good way to keep occupational activities from aggravating symptoms.

Psychological counseling. Talking to a psychologist or a therapist may help to manage the emotional stress that can exacerbate symptoms and may even help reduce the severity of symptoms. Some people with fibromyalgia are depressed by their efforts to cope with a disorder that causes chronic pain. Others may have major depression that requires the use of antidepressant medication. The need for psychological counseling is not a sign of weakness or mental instability, and it does not mean that a patient's symptoms are all "in their head." Rather, counseling can be valuable in helping

NEW RESEARCH

More Antibiotics May Not Help Lingering Lyme Disease

One round of antibiotics is enough to cure Lyme disease in most cases, but some people continue to experience fatigue and impaired thinking. Two new studies suggest that additional antibiotics do not help improve mental function, although one of the studies found that a second round of antibiotics may decrease fatigue.

The first study examined 129 people treated for Lyme disease who still had symptoms such as impaired thinking and severe fatigue. Participants were randomized to receive either intravenous ceftriaxone (Rocephin) for 30 days followed by oral doxycycline (Vibramycin) for 60 days, or a placebo. After 180 days, there were no differences in mental function between the groups.

The second study involved 55 people who had severe fatigue for at least six months after treatment for Lyme disease. They were randomized to receive 28 days of intravenous ceftriaxone or a placebo. Six months later, 64% of the ceftriaxone group had reduced fatigue, compared with 19% of the placebo group. The antibiotics had no effect on mental function. The authors point out that 7% of the participants had adverse reactions to the intravenous infusions that required hospitalization, and they conclude that they do not support the use of additional therapy with ceftriaxone.

NEUROLOGY
Volume 60, pages 1916 and 1923
June 24, 2003

The Benefits of Counseling for Fibromyalgia

Fibromyalgia is a physical condition, but treating related psychological distress may help reduce pain.

Because diagnostic tests reveal no visible abnormalities in people with fibromyalgia, many doctors once considered the condition to be a psychological problem. Today, fibromyalgia is known to be a physical disorder. However, it does have a psychological component: A painful flare-up of fibromyalgia can cause psychological distress, just as increased psychological distress can cause a flare-up.

People with fibromyalgia are more likely to suffer from psychological distress than either the general population or people with other types of chronic widespread pain. Approximately 20% to 30% of people with fibromyalgia are clinically depressed at any given time, and half of all people with fibromyalgia will experience anxiety or major depression at some point in their lives (compared with 10% to 20% of the general population).

Researchers have not been able to determine whether the pain and fatigue of fibromyalgia lead to psychological distress, or whether the same underlying factors cause both fibromyalgia and distress. Nonetheless, antidepressant medications are helpful in relieving pain in 30% to 50% of people with fibromyalgia. In addition, psychological counseling—particularly cognitive-behavioral therapy and group psychotherapy—can help some people with fibromyalgia. Both types of therapy teach patients how to reduce the psychological distress that both contributes to and results from their condition. The result is often improved daily functioning and reduced symptoms.

Cognitive-Behavioral Therapy

Cognitive-behavioral therapy is a type of counseling that teaches people to recognize their distorted views and change their destructive thought patterns and actions. Therapy is conducted with a therapist on an individual basis or in a group setting.

People with chronic illnesses such as fibromyalgia often develop distorted perceptions or patterns of thought that can contribute to their physical pain. For example, a person with fibromyalgia who needs to take a lot of sick days because of his condition might jump to the conclusion that he is a bad employee. Or a person might see her inability to control her fibromyalgia as evidence that she is a total failure. Cognitive-behavioral therapy helps people evaluate these incorrect perceptions and replace them with thoughts that reinforce their self-worth and competence.

Therapy sessions also involve teaching people skills such as relaxation techniques to help them cope with their physical limitations and ways to set realistic limits so that they can feel as successful as possible. These adaptations can help reduce the distress and symptoms associated with fibromyalgia.

A recent study in The Journal of Rheumatology compared 69 patients who received standard treatment for fibromyalgia (antidepressants, pain relievers, and exercise instruction) with 76 patients who received the standard treatment plus six sessions

to manage a chronic illness. For more information on psychological counseling for fibromyalgia, see the feature above.

Medication. Drug therapy for fibromyalgia can relieve pain and improve sleep. Since inflammation is not a part of this syndrome, corticosteroids or high doses of NSAIDs are not prescribed. However, judicious use of NSAIDs or acetaminophen (see pages 12–18) may provide pain relief during flares.

Abnormal sleep patterns typically are treated with low doses of tricyclic antidepressants, such as amitriptyline (Elavil and Endep), or nortriptyline (Aventyl and Pamelor). Doctors start patients on a dosage of about 10 mg of the tricyclic, taken one to two hours before bedtime, and then slowly raise the dose. It may take some time to find the optimal dosage. Antidepressant drugs called selective serotonin reuptake inhibitors, such as fluoxetine (Prozac) and sertraline (Zoloft), are another option. People should keep in mind that they of cognitive-behavioral therapy over a four-week period. The sessions included instruction on managing negative thoughts and attitudes, relaxing muscles, and improving function. Neither group had significant reductions in pain, but 25% of the cognitive-behavioral therapy group experienced improvements in daily functioning, compared with 12% of the standard therapy group. Although other studies have shown modest reductions in pain, the cognitive-behavioral therapy in this study was designed to improve physical function, rather than pain.

Group Psychotherapy

In group psychotherapy, 5 to 10 people, often with the same medical condition or emotional problem, meet together with a therapist once or twice a week. The discussion is guided by the therapist, who attempts to address the concerns of both individual members and the group as a whole. Participants are encouraged, but not required, to share their thoughts and feelings with the group and to comment on what other members say. Group psychotherapy for fibromyalgia may also include some elements of cognitive-behavioral therapy such as

instruction on controlling negative thoughts or reducing anxiety.

For people with fibromyalgia, group psychotherapy may be even more helpful than individual counseling sessions because of the support and feedback offered by other people dealing with the same problem. Fewer studies have been conducted on group psychotherapy than on cognitive-behavioral therapy, but some research suggests that it can help reduce some of the symptoms of fibromyalgia.

In one small study, 24 people with fibromyalgia participated in a one-year

outpatient treatment program and an eight-week course that taught coping skills. Another group of 35 patients received this treatment in addition to participating in a 90-minute group psychotherapy session once a week for 14 weeks. At the end of the study, the psychotherapy group reported less depression, morning and overall fatigue, and pain than they had at the beginning of the study. One theory is that by lessening isolation and creating a social support system that makes life more meaningful, group psychotherapy can reduce distress and fibromyalgia symptoms.

How To Find a Therapist
Your doctor may be able to recommend a cognitive-behavioral therapist or a group psychotherapist. Alternatively, the following organizations can direct you to a therapist in your area. (The American Psychological Association does not give referrals, but you can call the organization at 800-964-2000 to get contact information for a referral service in your area.)

National Association of Cognitive-Behavioral Therapists
P.O. Box 2195
Weirton, WV 26062
☎ 800-853-1135
www.nacbt.org

American Group Psychotherapy Association
26 East 21st Street, 6th Floor
New York, NY 10010
☎ 877-668-AGPA/212-477-2677
www.agpa.org

---

may take as long as four to six weeks to respond to drug therapy.

If people have severe pain in a specific area, injection of an anesthetic (usually procaine) can provide relief. Benefits are felt within two to five days and can last two to four months. However, injections can only be given every three months.

Bursitis

Bursitis is an inflammation of one of the small fluid-filled sacs, or bursae, that act as cushions in areas of the body where muscles or tendons move over bones or other muscles. Bursae prevent friction by protecting muscles and tendons from coming into direct contact with bones. When a bursa becomes inflamed, pain and swelling result. There are about 150 bursae in the body, but the ones most commonly affected are in the shoulders, elbows, hips, knees, and feet. While bursitis may produce some of the same symptoms as arthritis, it affects the tissues surrounding the joint rather than the joint itself. Bursitis is not chronic (most cases clear up by themselves within a few days to two weeks), but it can recur unless protective measures are adopted.

CAUSES OF BURSITIS

Bursitis can be caused by excessive pressure or by a bump, blow, or fall, but in most cases it results from joint overuse due to repetitive motions. Bursitis in the shoulder can be brought on by excessive strain (for example, from serving a tennis ball). Elbow bursitis most often results from a bump or blow or from frequently resting the elbow on a hard surface, such as a desk. Foot problems that cause improper alignment of the legs can irritate the bursae in the hips; one common cause is wearing shoes that have worn heels. Ill-fitting or uncomfortable shoes can cause a bunion—which is actually an inflammation of the bursa near the joint at the base of the big toe.

People with arthritis are at greater risk for developing bursitis because they may try to compensate for sore joints by making awkward or exaggerated movements that lead to improper body mechanics. Thus, everyday activities may irritate the bursae.

PREVENTION OF BURSITIS

The best way to prevent bursitis is to avoid activities that require repetitive motions, although this is not always possible. Staying in shape helps prevent bursitis, since well-conditioned muscles are less susceptible to overuse injuries than tight or weak muscles. Still, exercise must be done in moderation, and activity should be stopped immediately if pain occurs. Be sure to increase the pace or intensity of a workout gradually.

SYMPTOMS OF BURSITIS

The primary symptom of bursitis is pain in the affected area. In most cases, the pain is dull and persistent and increases with movement, but it can be severe enough to awaken the individual at night. Though localized, the pain may radiate down an arm or leg. The bursa may be swollen and tender. Redness and warmth indicate the bursa has become infected.

Anatomy of a Bursa

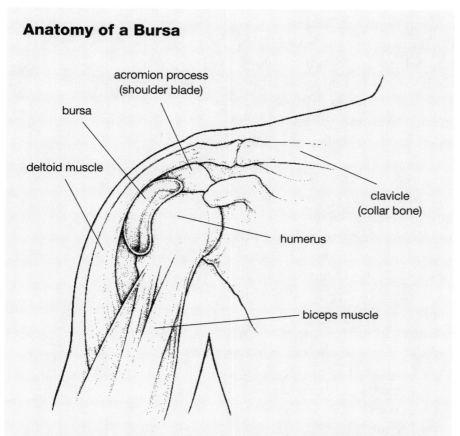

acromion process
(shoulder blade)

bursa

deltoid muscle

clavicle
(collar bone)

humerus

biceps muscle

Bursae are small, fluid-filled sacs that surround every joint and prevent friction where muscles cross bones or tendons. There are more than 150 bursae in the body. If a bursa becomes inflamed owing to strain or overuse, the condition is called bursitis. The illustration above shows a bursa in the shoulder, the area most commonly affected by bursitis.

DIAGNOSIS OF BURSITIS

A physical exam that includes inspection of the joint and surrounding tissues is the primary diagnostic method. The doctor will probably ask when the pain began, what makes the pain worse, if the onset of pain was related to any activity (particularly a new activity) or injury, if similar pain occurred in the past, and if any pain medications are being taken. Bursitis is not visible on x-rays, but sometimes an x-ray is taken to see if pain is caused by joint inflammation or some other cause.

TREATMENT OF BURSITIS

A suspected case of bursitis can be safely treated at home. The first step is to rest the affected area until the pain is gone, by eliminating or cutting back on the activity that brought on the problem. Apply ice packs to the affected area for 20 minutes every one to two hours to help reduce pain and swelling. (Applying ice for more than 20 minutes at a time can lead to frostbite.) After 48 hours, use heat to stimulate blood flow and help ease the pain. Aspirin or other NSAIDs can alleviate pain (see pages 13–18 and the chart on pages 16–17); acetaminophen is not effective for bursitis because it does not relieve inflammation.

After the pain subsides, do gentle stretching exercises and gradually build up to your usual level of activity. Do not massage the area, as this will only further irritate the bursa. Some people find liniments and ointments (fluids and creams that are applied to the skin to relieve pain and stiffness) to be helpful, although they do not repair the damage. Many of these products contain an ingredient that irritates the nerve endings in the skin and "confuses" the nervous system into feeling less intense pain.

If pain is disabling or does not subside after three or four days, consult a physician. In some instances, cortisone injections into the bursa can help reduce swelling and inflammation; this treatment is usually used for bursitis of the hip or shoulder. Another approach involves the removal of fluid from the bursa with a needle and syringe; this is usually used for bursitis of the elbow. In rare cases, surgery may be required to remove the troublesome bursa. ■

GLOSSARY

antimalarials—Drugs normally used to treat malaria but sometimes effective in the treatment of rheumatoid arthritis. The most commonly used antimalarial is hydroxychloroquine sulfate (Plaquenil).

arthroplasty—Implantation of a mechanical joint to replace a diseased or damaged joint. Also called total joint replacement surgery.

arthroscopy—A diagnostic and surgical technique that uses a thin tube with a light and tiny video camera at one end to view the inside of a joint.

articular cartilage—The cartilage that covers the ends of the bones.

autoimmune disorder—A disorder, such as rheumatoid arthritis, that results when the body's tissues are attacked by its own immune system.

bisphosphonate—A class of drugs used to maintain or improve bone density.

Bouchard's nodes—Knobby overgrowths of the middle joint of the fingers in people with osteoarthritis.

bursa—A small, fluid-filled sac between a tendon and a bone that protects muscles and tendons from coming into direct contact with bones.

bursitis—Inflammation of a bursa, especially in the shoulder, elbow, hip, knee, or foot.

cartilage—The connective tissue that covers the ends of bones and acts as the body's shock absorber by cushioning the bones from weight-bearing stress. Contains water, chondrocytes, collagen, and proteoglycans.

chondrocyte—A cartilage cell.

collagen—The major protein of connective tissue, cartilage, and bone.

coronary heart disease—A narrowing of the coronary arteries that results in inadequate blood flow to the heart.

corticosteroids—Potent drugs that are used to reduce the pain and inflammation associated with rheumatoid arthritis and other autoimmune disorders. Also called steroids.

cyclooxygenase-2 (COX-2) inhibitors—Anti-inflammatory drugs that work by blocking the COX-2 enzyme, which plays a role in inflammation, but not the COX-1 enzyme, which helps protect the digestive tract.

cytoprotective drugs—Medications that decrease the acid content of the stomach, reducing the risk of developing an ulcer when taking NSAIDs.

disease-modifying antirheumatic drugs (DMARDs)—Anti-inflammatory drugs that not only help relieve the pain and inflammation of rheumatoid arthritis but also slow the progression of the disease. Once considered a treatment of last resort, they are now prescribed earlier in the course of the disease.

disease-modifying osteoarthritis drugs (DMOADs)—A class of medications aimed at preventing joint damage in people with osteoarthritis by inhibiting the release of enzymes that break down cartilage. Thus far, no agent has been shown to have this effect in humans.

fibromyalgia syndrome—A rheumatic disorder characterized by body aches, pain, stiffness, sleep disturbances, and fatigue, as well as tenderness in specific sites on the body. Occurs predominately in women.

gout—A disease characterized by increased blood levels of uric acid that produces pain and inflammation in the joints, particularly in the foot, ankle, or knee.

Heberden's nodes—Knobby overgrowths of the joint nearest the fingertips in people with osteoarthritis.

hyperuricemia—Excess uric acid in the blood.

immunosuppressant—A medication that suppresses the body's immune response.

joint capsule—A sac-like envelope that encloses a joint. Consists of an inner synovial membrane and an outer fibrous membrane.

ligament—A band of fibrous tissue that connects two bones.

meniscal cartilage—Fibrous cartilage that acts as an additional shock absorber between the bones of the knee.

nonsteroidal anti-inflammatory drugs (NSAIDs)—Medications that relieve joint pain and stiffness by reducing inflammation. Some examples are aspirin and ibuprofen.

osteoarthritis (OA)—A type of arthritis characterized by pain and stiffness in the joints, such as those in the hands, hips, knees, spine, or feet, due to breakdown of cartilage.

pannus—A thickening of the synovial membrane resulting from an overgrowth of synovial cells and an accumulation of white blood cells. Occurs as rheumatoid arthritis progresses.

podagra—Severe pain in the big toe caused by gout.

primary osteoarthritis—The gradual breakdown of cartilage that occurs with age and is due to stress on a joint.

proteoglycans—Components of cartilage that help absorb the shock of body movements and provide the joints with strength and elasticity.

purine—A substance that can be converted to uric acid in the body.

rheumatoid arthritis—A chronic autoimmune disease characterized by pain, stiffness, inflammation, swelling, and, sometimes, destruction of joints.

secondary osteoarthritis—Osteoarthritis that results from trauma to the joint or from chronic joint injury due to another type of arthritis, such as rheumatoid arthritis.

slow-acting antirheumatic drugs (SAARDs)—See **disease-modifying antirheumatic drugs (DMARDs).**

synovectomy—Removal of the synovial membrane from a joint.

synovial fluid—A lubricating fluid secreted by the synovial membrane.

synovial membrane—Connective tissue that lines the cavity of a joint and produces synovial fluid.

systemic lupus erythematosus (SLE)—An inflammatory disease of connective tissue that is characterized by skin rash, arthritis, and inflammation of different organs. Occurs primarily in women.

tidal irrigation—A treatment for osteoarthritis of the knee in which a saline solution is repeatedly injected into and then withdrawn from the joint space to remove debris from the joint and help break up the synovial membrane that has adhered to itself.

tophi—Deposits of uric acid crystals in the skin or around joints.

trigger point—A specific spot on the body that will elicit pain if touched in people with fibromyalgia.

tumor necrosis factor—A protein that plays an early and major role in the rheumatic disease process.

viscosupplementation—A treatment option for people with osteoarthritis of the knee that involves the injection of hyaluronan, a natural component of synovial fluid, directly into the knee joint.

HEALTH INFORMATION ORGANIZATIONS AND SUPPORT GROUPS

**American Academy of
Orthopaedic Surgeons**
6300 N. River Rd.
Rosemont, IL 60018-4262
☎ 800-824-BONES
www.aaos.org
Professional organization concerned
with skeletal deformities. Publishes
information on orthopedic disorders;
see their Web site or call for
information.

Arthritis Foundation
P.O. Box 7669
Atlanta, GA 30357-0669
☎ 800-283-7800/404-872-7100
www.arthritis.org
Provides information about causes,
symptoms, diagnosis, and treatment of
arthritis; offers support groups and
supports arthritis research.

The Arthritis Society
393 University Ave., Ste. 1700
Toronto, Ontario
M5G 1E6 Canada
☎ 416-979-7228
www.arthritis.ca
Not-for-profit organization dedicated
to finding the cause of (and ultimately
the cure for) arthritis. Publishes
information pamphlets and videos.

Lupus Foundation of America
2000 L St. NW, Ste. 710
Washington, DC 20036
☎ 800-558-0121/202-349-1155
www.lupus.org
Nationwide charitable foundation that
provides support groups and seeks
funding for ongoing research.

**National Institute of Arthritis &
Musculoskeletal & Skin Diseases
Information Clearinghouse**
National Institutes of Health
One AMS Circle
Bethesda, MD 20892-3675
☎ 877-226-4267/301-495-4484
www.niams.nih.gov
A branch of the NIH. Provides
information about diseases of the
bone, joint, muscle, and skin.

LEADING HOSPITALS

U.S. News & World Report and the National Opinion Research Center, a social-science research group at the University of Chicago, recently conducted their 14th annual nationwide survey of 8,160 physicians in 17 medical specialties. The doctors nominated up to five hospitals they consider best from among 6,003 U.S. hospitals. These are the current lists of the best hospitals for orthopedics and rheumatology, as determined by the doctors' recommendations from 2001, 2002, and 2003; federal data on death rates; and factual data regarding quality indicators, such as the ratio of registered nurses to patients and the use of advanced technology. Since the results reflect the doctors' opinions, they are subjective to some degree. Any institution listed is considered a leading center, and the rankings do not imply that other hospitals cannot or do not deliver excellent care.

ORTHOPEDIC MEDICINE

1. **Mayo Clinic,** Rochester, MN
2. **Hospital for Special Surgery,** New York, NY
3. **Massachusetts General Hospital,** Boston, MA
4. **Johns Hopkins Hospital,** Baltimore, MD
5. **Cleveland Clinic,** Cleveland, OH
6. **Duke University Medical Center,** Durham, NC
7. **University of California, Los Angeles Medical Center,** Los Angeles, CA
8. **University of Iowa Hospitals and Clinics,** Iowa City, IA
9. **Harborview Medical Center,** Seattle, WA
10. **University of Washington Medical Center,** Seattle, WA

RHEUMATOLOGY

1. **Mayo Clinic,** Rochester, MN
2. **Johns Hopkins Hospital,** Baltimore, MD
3. **Hospital for Special Surgery,** New York, NY
4. **Cleveland Clinic,** Cleveland, OH
5. **University of California, Los Angeles Medical Center,** Los Angeles, CA
6. **University of Alabama Hospital,** Birmingham, AL
7. **Massachusetts General Hospital,** Boston, MA
8. **Brigham and Women's Hospital,** Boston, MA
9. **Duke University Medical Center,** Durham, NC
10. **University of California, San Francisco Medical Center,** San Francisco, CA

© *U.S. News & World Report,* July 28, 2003.

OBESITY AND HIP REPLACEMENT

Doctors have known for some time that excess body weight increases a person's odds of developing osteoarthritis of the knee, but evidence had not clearly linked excess weight to osteoarthritis of the hip. Now, researchers have found that obesity—particularly at a young age—increases the risk of hip osteoarthritis.

In the study reprinted here from *The American Journal of Medicine,* researchers led by Elizabeth W. Karlson, M.D., of Brigham and Women's Hospital in Boston, analyzed data from the Nurses' Health Study. This study has followed more than 121,000 nurses (age 30 to 55 at entry) since 1976. The researchers determined that women with a current body mass index (BMI; a ratio of weight to height) of 35 or greater were two times more likely to have had a hip replacement because of severe hip osteoarthritis than women with the lowest BMIs (less than 22).

And obesity was even more detrimental at a young age than later in life. In fact, women with BMIs of 35 or greater at age 18 (based on self-reports) had more than five times the risk of a hip replacement than those with BMIs below 22 at that age. In addition, any increase in BMI over 22 was linked to an increased risk of hip replacement. (To calculate your BMI, multiply your weight in pounds by 703 and divide that number by your height in inches squared. People with a BMI of 25 or more are overweight. A BMI of 30 or more indicates obesity, and those with a BMI of 35 or higher have severe obesity.)

These data indicate that the risk of osteoarthritis-related hip replacement is established early in the life of obese people, possibly because obesity alters the way people walk. Furthermore, becoming obese at an early age increases the number of years that the hip is subjected to the excess weight.

The research also revealed that other modifiable risk factors for osteoarthritis—including exercise, smoking, alcohol consumption, and the use of hormone replacement therapy—did not affect the risk of hip replacement. However, age did have an effect: Women age 70 or older had nine times as many hip replacements as women younger than age 55.

Total Hip Replacement Due to Osteoarthritis: The Importance of Age, Obesity, and Other Modifiable Risk Factors

Elizabeth W. Karlson, MD, Lisa A. Mandl, MD, MPH, Gideon N. Aweh, MS, Oliver Sangha†, MD, ScD, Matthew H. Liang, MD, MPH, Francine Grodstein, ScD

PURPOSE: We studied whether several modifiable factors were associated with the risk of total hip replacement due to hip osteoarthritis among women.

METHODS: We identified 568 women from the Nurses' Health Study who reported total hip replacement due to primary hip osteoarthritis on questionnaires from 1990 to 1996, using a validated algorithm. The relation of potential risk factors, such as age, body mass index, physical activity, smoking, alcohol intake, and hormone use, to hip replacement was assessed using pooled logistic regression models.

RESULTS: Higher body mass index was associated with an increased risk of hip replacement due to osteoarthritis (P for trend = 0.0001). Compared with women in the lowest category of body mass index (<22 kg/m^2), those in the highest category of body mass index (≥ 35 kg/m^2) had a twofold increased risk (95% confidence interval [CI]: 1.4 to 2.8), whereas those in the highest category of body mass index at age 18 years had more than a fivefold increased risk (95% CI: 2.5 to 10.7). Age also had a positive association; women aged ≥ 70 years were nine times more likely to have hip replacement than those aged <55 years (95% CI: 5.4 to 13.9). Recreational physical activity, smoking, alcohol use, and postmenopausal hormone use were not associated with an increased risk of hip replacement.

CONCLUSION: In the Nurses' Health Study, higher body mass index and older age significantly increased the risk of total hip replacement due to osteoarthritis. Part of this risk appeared to be established early in life. **Am J Med. 2003;114:93–98.** ©2003 by Excerpta Medica Inc.

Osteoarthritis is the most common form of chronic arthritis and results in more functional loss than any other disease, including heart disease and cancer (1). In the United States, its economic impact has been estimated at $15.5 billion (in 1994) (2). Although potentially modifiable risk factors, such as obesity, have been associated with osteoarthritis of the knee (3–9), the relation with hip osteoarthritis is unclear. For example, several studies have suggested that obesity increases the risk of symptomatic (10–18) but not radiographic hip osteoarthritis (3,19). Furthermore, because most studies have been cross-sectional (9–11,13–15, 17,20), it is not known if obesity preceded or followed hip pathology, because symptoms may lead patients to limit activity and gain weight.

Thus, we studied whether modifiable risk factors such as body mass index, postmenopausal hormone use, physical activity, or cigarette smoking were related to hip osteoarthritis that was severe enough to warrant total hip replacement in a large, prospective cohort of women.

METHODS

The Nurses' Health Study is a prospective cohort of 121,701 female nurses who were aged 30 to 55 years in 1976. Information on diseases, lifestyle, and health practices is collected from the subjects via biennial questionnaires, with a response rate of greater than 90% for each questionnaire.

We used self-reported total hip replacement on the 1990 to 1996 questionnaires as a surrogate for clinically severe primary hip osteoarthritis. We mailed a supplementary questionnaire to all participants who reported a hip replacement, which asked about the date of surgery, the diagnosis of osteoarthritis, and other conditions (e.g., major hip trauma, fracture, congenital dysplasia, osteonecrosis, or inflammatory arthritis) that led to hip replacement. Primary hip osteoarthritis was defined as hip replacement, without the presence of these other conditions.

The questionnaire was validated by reviewing preoperative radiographs from randomly selected women, of whom 100 reported primary osteoarthritis and 50 reported other reasons for hip replacement. The response rate was 56% (n = 84) after three mailings, and 60 radiographs were interpretable. Two radiologists who were

From the Division of Rheumatology, Immunology, and Allergy, Robert B. Brigham Arthritis and Musculoskeletal Diseases Clinical Research Center, Channing Laboratory, Department of Medicine, Brigham and Women's Hospital, Harvard Medical School, Boston, Massachusetts.

†Deceased. Formerly from the University of Munich, School of Medicine.

Supported by grants AR42630, CA87969, AR36308, and K08 AR 02074-1 from the National Institutes of Health, Bethesda, Maryland. Dr. Karlson is the recipient of an Arthritis Foundation Investigator Award. Dr. Mandl is a recipient of an Arthritis Foundation Physician Scientist Award.

Requests for reprints should be addressed to Elizabeth W. Karlson, MD, 75 Francis Street, Boston, Massachusetts 02115, or ekarlson@partners.org.

Manuscript submitted January 29, 2002, and accepted in revised form August 22, 2002.

blinded to diagnosis reviewed the radiographs. Ninety-three percent (41/44) of women who reported primary osteoarthritis had this diagnosis confirmed by radiographs, 80% (35/44) had a radiographic severity of grade 3 or higher on the Kellgren-Lawrence scale, and only 7% (3/44) had radiographic evidence of other diagnoses (either osteonecrosis or congenital hip dysplasia). Of 16 women who reported secondary osteoarthritis (e.g., due to congenital hip dysplasia, osteonecrosis or inflammatory arthritis), the diagnosis was confirmed by radiograph in 13 (81%). Thus, in this cohort of nurses, self-reported hip replacement and a report of hip osteoarthritis identified clinically important primary hip osteoarthritis reliably and with minimal misclassification.

Subjects

We excluded women who did not respond in 1990 (the baseline in our study), prevalent cases of hip replacement in 1990, women who indicated secondary reasons for hip replacement, and nonresponders to the supplementary questionnaire. We also excluded women with self-reported rheumatoid arthritis, hip fracture, cancer, or, in particular, cardiovascular disease, which is strongly associated with body mass index and may have been a contraindication for elective hip replacement surgery. Thus, the final sample included 93,442 women followed from 1990 to 1996.

Exposures

Body mass index was computed for each 2-year interval using the weight in kilograms divided by height in meters squared reported at cohort entry in 1976 (when the mean [± SD] age was 42.9 ± 7.2 years) and categorized as <22 kg/m^2 (reference group), 22 to 24.9 kg/m^2, 25 to 29.9 kg/m^2, 30 to 34.9 kg/m^2, or ≥35 kg/m^2. Body mass index at age 18 years was calculated using weight at that age (collected in 1980) and height reported in 1976. In a validation study that compared self-reported weight with direct measurement, the correlation coefficient was R = 0.96 (21). Self-reported weight at age 18 years was also strongly correlated with weight recorded in medical records in a similar cohort of nurses (R = 0.87) (22).

We defined physical activity as the cumulative average level of recreational activity (e.g., walking, hiking, running, aerobics). We averaged the hours per week of moderate or vigorous physical activity for each follow-up period from 1990 to 1996 and categorized physical activity as <1, 1 to 1.9, 2 to 3.9, 4 to 6.9, or ≥7 hours per week. The questionnaire does not contain data on occupational activity or physical workload, both of which have been associated with hip osteoarthritis (13,14,18,23–25).

Postmenopausal hormone use was categorized as current, past, or never. Smoking was categorized as never, past, or current (0 to 14, 15 to 24, or ≥25 cigarettes per day). Information on oral contraceptive use was collected from 1976 to 1982 (after which the cohort was aged 36 to

61 years and use was uncommon). Parity, defined as 0, 1, 2, 3, or ≥4 children, was assessed through 1984 (after which the cohort was aged 38 to 63 years and childbirth was uncommon). Alcohol use (e.g., wine, beer, liquor) was ascertained every 4 years on a food frequency questionnaire and categorized as 0, <5, 5 to 9, 10 to 14, or ≥15 g/d.

Statistical Analysis

We used logistic regression models to study the association between hip replacement due to osteoarthritis and the following risk factors: age (<55, 55 to 59, 60 to 64, 65 to 69, or ≥70 years), body mass index, recreational physical activity, smoking, alcohol intake, past oral contraceptive use, postmenopausal hormone use, and parity. A secondary analysis examined the effect of weight change (10-kg weight loss, ± 10 kg, >10-kg weight gain) since age 18 years. All variables were time varying, and data were updated using information from the biennial questionnaires starting at baseline in 1990. Consequently, each subject contributed person-time of follow-up from the time of the questionnaire to the end of the follow-up period, the date of the first hip replacement, death, or loss due to follow-up, whichever came first. Relative risks and 95% confidence intervals were estimated. Since women may have changed their behavior after the onset of hip pain, in alternate analyses we stopped updating data on body mass index, physical activity, and smoking on the date of self-reported first hip symptoms. Results of these analyses were identical; thus, only results from the primary analysis are presented. All analyses were performed using SAS software, Version 8 (SAS Institute Inc., Cary, North Carolina).

RESULTS

Of the 1435 women who reported hip replacement from 1990 to 1996, 1142 (80%) responded to the supplemental questionnaire to confirm the diagnosis of primary osteoarthritis. Of these, 871 women (76%) reported hip replacement due to osteoarthritis. We excluded 137 women who had surgery before 1990 and 166 who had cancer or cardiovascular disease, leaving 568 cases for analysis.

Women with higher body mass index were less likely to take postmenopausal hormones, exercise, drink alcohol, or smoke than were women with lower body mass index (Table 1). The relative risk of hip replacement increased greatly with age (P for trend = 0.0001). After adjusting for confounding factors, women aged ≥70 years were almost nine times more likely to have a hip replacement than those younger than 55 years (95% confidence interval [CI]: 5.4 to 13.9; Table 2). Higher body mass index was also associated with an increased relative risk of hip replacement (P for trend = 0.0001). In multivariate-adjusted analyses, those in the highest category of body mass

Table 1. Age-Standardized Baseline Characteristics of Study Participants by Body Mass Index

Characteristic	Body Mass Index (kg/m^2)				
	<22 (n = 20,750)	22–24.9 (n = 27,746)	25–29.9 (n = 28,935)	30–34.9 (n = 10,940)	≥35 (n = 4964)
	Number (%) or Mean ± SD				
Premenopausal	4565 (22)	6104 (22)	6076 (21)	2407 (22)	1092 (22)
Ever used oral contraceptive pills	10,583 (51)	13,596 (41)	13,599 (47)	4923 (45)	2234 (45)
Ever used postmenopausal hormones	9545 (46)	12,486 (45)	11,863 (41)	4048 (37)	1489 (30)
Parity	19,298 (93)	25,804 (93)	27,199 (94)	10,284 (94)	4617 (93)
Recreational activity >7 hours per week	2905 (14)	3330 (12)	2894 (10)	875 (8)	347 (7)
Current smoker	4773 (23)	5272 (19)	5272 (16)	1422 (13)	496 (10)
Alcohol intake (g/d)	4.9 ± 9.5	4.4 ± 8.9	3.4 ± 8.1	2.3 ± 6.7	1.6 ± 5.7

index (≥35 kg/m^2) had almost a threefold greater risk than those in the lowest category of body mass index (22 kg/m^2) (Table 3). In an analysis of body mass index at age 18 years that excluded recent body mass index, body mass index was associated strongly with an increased relative risk of hip replacement. All relative risks for body mass index at age 18 years were significantly greater than those in analyses that included recent body mass index, and the relative risk rose to 7.4 (95% CI: 3.6 to 15.0) when the highest and lowest categories were compared (Table 3). When we included both recent body mass index and body mass index at age 18 years in a model, the relative risks for each were only somewhat attenuated (Table 3).

To investigate whether the risk due to body mass index at age 18 years was due to subsequent weight change, we adjusted for the difference in weight at entry and at age 18 years and still found an increase in the risk of hip replacement with higher body mass index. For example, the relative risk was 7.5 (95% CI: 3.5 to 16.0) when the highest and lowest categories of body mass index at age 18 years were compared. A weight gain of more than 10 kg from 1976 to the date of hip replacement was associated with a modest increase in the risk of hip replacement (relative risk [RR] = 1.2; 95% CI: 1.0 to 1.5). Weight loss of more than 10 kg did not appear to have protective effects (RR = 1.1; 95% CI: 0.7 to 1.8); however, few women lost weight.

We found no significant association between hip replacement due to osteoarthritis and other modifiable risk factors, including moderate-to-vigorous recreational physical activity, oral contraceptive use, current or past postmenopausal hormone use, parity, alcohol use, or smoking (Table 2).

DISCUSSION

In a cohort of more than 93,000 female nurses, we found that high body mass index was a risk factor for total hip replacement due to osteoarthritis. In addition, a substantial risk associated with body mass index was established early in life; even modest increments in body mass index

at age 18 years were associated with a greater risk of future hip replacement. Unlike some studies (17,20,26–30), we found no association between hip replacement due to osteoarthritis and postmenopausal hormone therapy, smoking, or recreational activity. Although weight gain of more than 10 kg after the age of 18 years seemed to increase the risk established early in life by 20%, we were unable to demonstrate that weight loss was protective, which had been shown in the Framingham study (5) for risk of symptomatic knee osteoarthritis, probably because only a few women with hip replacement had lost weight.

Many studies of knee osteoarthritis have established that body mass index is an important risk factor (3–9). However, results from epidemiologic studies of the risk of obesity and radiographic hip osteoarthritis have been inconsistent, with some suggesting no association (3,19), one demonstrating an association only with bilateral radiographic hip osteoarthritis (13), and others reporting sex (11) and race (10) differences in the association. In another study (30), women older than 65 years with moderate-to-severe hip osteoarthritis reported a higher body mass index at age 25 years than did those without hip osteoarthritis.

All of these studies, however, focused on radiographic osteoarthritis. Since only 40% to 50% of patients with radiographic osteoarthritis report pain, the determinants of symptomatic hip osteoarthritis may be different from those defined by radiograph alone (31,32). With one exception (33), several retrospective or cross-sectional studies of symptomatic hip osteoarthritis support a modest association with increased body mass index (9,12,14–17,20). In addition, two studies (12,16) suggested that body mass index in early life is a stronger predictor of hip replacement than more recent body mass index; however, these studies were cross-sectional and substantially smaller than our study. In a cohort of male physicians (34), being overweight at a younger age (20 to 29 years) was associated with symptomatic knee osteoarthritis but not symptomatic hip osteoarthritis later in life. However,

Table 2. Relative Risk of Total Hip Replacement Due to Osteoarthritis, by Age and Modifiable Factors

Risk Factor	No. with Hip Replacement*	Person-Years	Relative Risk[†] (95% Confidence Interval)
Age (years)			
<55	34	220,783	Reference
55–59	78	146,262	2.9 (1.8–4.5)
60–64	146	137,182	5.6 (3.6–8.7)
65–69	211	123,906	9.1 (5.9–14.0)
≥70	99	54,619	8.7 (5.4–13.9)
Oral contraceptive use			
Never	358	343,087	Reference
Past	204	319,188	1.0 (0.8–1.2)
Postmenopausal hormone use[‡]			
Never	176	179,555	Reference
Past	150	107,882	1.2 (1.0–1.5)
Current	189	234,682	1.0 (0.8–1.2)
Parity			
0	40	44,487	Reference
1	31	48,109	0.8 (0.5–1.3)
2	133	188,201	1.0 (0.7–1.4)
3	154	184,865	1.0 (0.7–1.4)
≥4	202	208,435	1.0 (0.7–1.4)
Physical activity (hours per week)			
<1	99	109,301	Reference
1–1.9	139	138,727	1.2 (0.9–1.5)
2–3.9	170	187,531	1.0 (0.8–1.3)
4–6.9	88	113,799	0.9 (0.7–1.3)
≥7	35	36,294	1.2 (0.8–1.7)
Alcohol (g/d)			
0	187	209,675	Reference
<5	155	171,609	1.1 (0.8–1.6)
5–9	36	52,643	0.5 (0.2–1.0)
10–14	46	43,398	1.4 (0.9–2.4)
≥15	55	47,619	1.5 (0.9–2.4)
Smoking			
Never	154	300,412	Reference
Past	178	212,331	1.2 (1.0–1.5)
Current (cigarettes per day)			
0–14	18	31,589	0.9 (0.6–1.5)
15–24	21	46,105	0.8 (0.5–1.3)
≥25	3	7455	0.8 (0.3–2.6)

* There was missing information on physical activity (n = 37 women), smoking (n = 194), alcohol (n = 89), postmenopausal hormone use (n = 40), oral contraceptive use (n = 6), and parity (n = 8).
[†] Adjusted for physical activity, smoking, alcohol, postmenopausal hormone use, oral contraceptive use, parity, body mass index at age 18 years, and current body mass index.
[‡] Limited to women who were postmenopausal at date of total hip replacement.

there were only 26 men with hip osteoarthritis. A recent study demonstrated an association between body mass index and subsequent hip replacement due to osteoarthritis in 268 men and 382 women, with a relative risk of 3.0 (95% CI: 2.1 to 4.1) for women in the highest body mass index group (≥27 kg/m^2) (18).

There are limited biologic data to support a relation between body mass index and hip osteoarthritis. Accelerated hip osteoarthritis can be produced surgically in an animal model (young dogs) by forcing the hips into ex-aggerated femoral anteversion (35). Similarly in humans, excess fat in the thighs may cause femoral anteversion during development. Studies comparing the walking gait of obese adults (36) and children (37,38) with that of nonobese subjects have demonstrated differences in mean hip abduction angles, gait symmetry, stride width, and dynamic stability, suggesting biomechanical effects of obesity on gait.

Our study has several limitations. The diagnosis of primary osteoarthritis was based on self-reported hip re-

Table 3. Relative Risk of Total Hip Replacement Due to Osteoarthritis, by Body Mass Index and Body Mass Index at Age 18 Years

Risk Factor	No. with Hip Replacement	Person-Years*	Relative Risk (95% Confidence Interval)
Body mass index[†] (kg/m²)			
<22	90	134,829	Reference
22–24.9	117	191,393	0.9 (0.7–1.2)
25–29.9	201	222,385	1.3 (1.0–1.7)
30–34.9	91	90,681	1.5 (1.1–2.0)
≥35	67	42,702	2.6 (1.9–3.6)
Body mass index[‡] (kg/m²)			
<22	90	134,829	Reference
22–24.9	117	191,393	0.9 (0.7–1.2)
25–29.9	201	222,385	1.2 (0.9–1.6)
30–34.9	91	90,681	1.3 (0.9–1.8)
≥35	67	42,702	2.0 (1.4–2.8)
Body mass index at age 18 years[†] (kg/m²)			
<22	284	403,900	Reference
22–24.9	133	126,416	1.5 (1.2–1.8)
25–29.9	64	45,141	2.0 (1.5–2.7)
30–34.9	15	8372	2.5 (1.5–4.3)
≥35	8	1472	7.4 (3.6–15.0)
Body mass index at age 18 years[§] (kg/m²)			
<22	284	403,900	Reference
22–24.9	133	126,416	1.3 (1.1–1.7)
25–29.9	64	45,141	1.7 (1.3–2.3)
30–34.9	15	8372	1.9 (1.1–3.3)
≥35	8	1472	5.2 (2.5–10.7)

* There was missing information on body mass index at age 18 years for 64 women and on current body mass index for 2 women.

[†] Adjusted for age, physical activity, smoking, alcohol, postmenopausal hormone use, oral contraceptive use, and parity.

[‡] Adjusted for age, physical activity, smoking, alcohol, postmenopausal hormone use, oral contraceptive use, parity, and body mass index at 18 years.

[§] Adjusted for age, physical activity, smoking, alcohol, postmenopausal hormone use, oral contraceptive use, parity, and current body mass index.

placement and diagnoses. However, the subjects are registered nurses with knowledge about health, and our validation study comparing radiographic diagnosis with self-report showed high accuracy. In addition, hip replacement reflects advanced osteoarthritis and the decision to proceed with surgery, therefore incorporating patient preference, access, and other factors that we did not measure. Some surgeons may have preferred not to operate on older or severely obese patients, which would have led to underestimation of the effect of older age or high body mass index. We did not have information on the history of injuries from all subjects or physical workload, both of which are possible risk factors (13,14,18,23–25). Because we only examined risk factors for clinically severe osteoarthritis leading to hip replacement, we could not distinguish between exposures that affected the risk of disease development and those that affected progression from mild to severe disease. Furthermore, we were unable to identify women with mild hip osteoarthritis, or hip osteoarthritis without hip replacement, who could have been included in the control group. Thus, our relative risk estimates may somewhat underestimate the true effects of age and body mass index if they are also risk factors for less severe hip osteoarthritis. Finally, our cohort was composed of female nurses who were similar in race, socioeconomic status, and education. However, many of the exposure and disease associations reported from the Nurses' Health Study are consistent with those in studies involving more heterogeneous samples, and it is unlikely that the biological relations among women in this cohort differ from women in general.

In conclusion, we found an increasing risk of total hip replacement due to osteoarthritis with older age and higher body mass index. The relation with body mass index was strongly apparent at age 18 years, suggesting that the risk is partly established at a younger age. Our data suggest the importance of interventions to reduce obesity, particularly at younger ages, to decrease morbidity and health care costs related to total joint replacement due to osteoarthritis.

ACKNOWLEDGMENT

We wish to thank the dedicated nurses in the Nurses' Health Study who have now participated in the study for more than 25 years. We also thank Julie Herbstman for her assistance, Drs. Piran Aliabadi and John Carrino for reviewing the radiographs, and Dr. Jeffrey Katz for reviewing the manuscript.

REFERENCES

1. Guccione AA, Felson DT, Anderson JJ, et al. The effects of specific medical conditions on the functional limitations of elders in the Framingham Study. *Am J Public Health.* 1994;84:351–358.

2. Yelin E. The economics of osteoarthritis. In: Brandt K, Doherty M, Lohmander SL, eds. *Osteoarthritis.* New York, New York: Oxford University Press; 1998:23–30.

3. Kellgren JH. Osteoarthritis in patients and populations. *BMJ.* 1961; 2:5243–5248.

4. Anderson JJ, Felson DT. Factors associated with osteoarthritis of the knee in the first national Health and Nutrition Examination Survey (HANES I). Evidence for an association with overweight, race, and physical demands of work. *Am J Epidemiol.* 1988;128: 179–189.

5. Felson DT, Zhang Y, Anthony JM, et al. Weight loss reduces the risk for symptomatic knee osteoarthritis in women. The Framingham Study. *Ann Intern Med.* 1992;116:535–539.

6. Felson DT, Zhang Y, Hannan MT, et al. The incidence and natural history of knee osteoarthritis in the elderly. The Framingham Osteoarthritis Study. *Arthritis Rheum.* 1995;38:1500–1505.

7. Felson DT, Zhang Y, Hannan MT, et al. Risk factors for incident radiographic knee osteoarthritis in the elderly: the Framingham Study. *Arthritis Rheum.* 1997;40:728–733.

8. Hart DJ, Doyle DV, Spector TD. Incidence and risk factors for radiographic knee osteoarthritis in middle-aged women: the Chingford Study. *Arthritis Rheum.* 1999;42:17–24.

9. Oliveria SA, Felson DT, Cirillo PA, et al. Body weight, body mass index, and incident symptomatic osteoarthritis of the hand, hip, and knee. *Epidemiology.* 1999;10:161–166.

10. Hartz AJ, Fischer ME, Bril G, et al. The association of obesity with joint pain and osteoarthritis in the HANES data. *J Chronic Dis.* 1986;39:311–319.

11. van Saase JL, Vandenbroucke JP, van Romunde LK, Valkenburg HA. Osteoarthritis and obesity in the general population. A relationship calling for an explanation. *J Rheumatol.* 1988;15:1152–1158.

12. Vingard E. Overweight predisposes to coxarthrosis. Body-mass index studied in 239 males with hip arthroplasty. *Acta Orthop Scand.* 1991;62:106–109.

13. Tepper S, Hochberg MC. Factors associated with hip osteoarthritis: data from the First National Health and Nutrition Examination Survey (NHANES-I). *Am J Epidemiol.* 1993;137:1081–1088.

14. Heliovaara M, Makela M, Impivaara O, et al. Association of overweight, trauma and workload with coxarthrosis. A health survey of 7,217 persons. *Acta Orthop Scand.* 1993;64:513–518.

15. Roach KE, Persky V, Miles T, Budiman-Mak E. Biomechanical aspects of occupation and osteoarthritis of the hip: a case-control study. *J Rheumatol.* 1994;21:2334–2340.

16. Vingard E, Alfredsson L, Malchau H. Lifestyle factors and hip arthrosis. A case referent study of body mass index, smoking and hormone therapy in 503 Swedish women. *Acta Orthop Scand.* 1997; 68:216–220.

17. Cooper C, Inskip H, Croft P, et al. Individual risk factors for hip osteoarthritis: obesity, hip injury, and physical activity. *Am J Epidemiol.* 1998;147:516–522.

18. Flugsrud GB, Nordsletten L, Espehaug B, et al. Risk factors for total hip replacement due to primary osteoarthritis: a cohort study in 50,034 persons. *Arthritis Rheum.* 2002;46:675–682.

19. Goldin RH, McAdam L, Louie JS, et al. Clinical and radiological survey of the incidence of osteoarthrosis among obese patients. *Ann Rheum Dis.* 1976;35:349–353.

20. Kraus JF, D'Ambrosia RD, Smith EG, et al. An epidemiological study of severe osteoarthritis. *Orthopedics.* 1978;1:37–42.

21. Willett W, Stampfer MJ, Bain C, et al. Cigarette smoking, relative weight, and menopause. *Am J Epidemiol.* 1983;117:651–658.

22. Troy LM, Hunter DJ, Manson JE, et al. The validity of recalled weight among younger women. *Int J Obes Relat Metab Disord.* 1995; 19:570–572.

23. Vingard E, Hogstedt C, Alfredsson L, et al. Coxarthrosis and physical work load. *Scand J Work Environ Health.* 1991;17:104–109.

24. Vingard E, Alfredsson L, Malchau H. Osteoarthrosis of the hip in women and its relation to physical load at work and in the home. *Ann Rheum Dis.* 1997;56:293–298.

25. Coggon D, Kellingray S, Inskip H, et al. Osteoarthritis of the hip and occupational lifting. *Am J Epidemiol.* 1998;147:523–528.

26. Spector TD, Hart DJ, Brown P, et al. Frequency of osteoarthritis in hysterectomized women. *J Rheumatol.* 1991;18:1877–1883.

27. Samanta A, Jones A, Regan M, et al. Is osteoarthritis in women affected by hormonal changes or smoking? *Br J Rheumatol.* 1993; 32:366–370.

28. Vingard E, Alfredsson L, Goldie I, Hogstedt C. Sports and osteoarthrosis of the hip. An epidemiologic study. *Am J Sports Med.* 1993; 21:195–200.

29. Nevitt MC, Cummings SR, Lane NE, et al. Association of estrogen replacement therapy with the risk of osteoarthritis of the hip in elderly white women. Study of Osteoporotic Fractures Research Group. *Arch Intern Med.* 1996;156:2073–2080.

30. Lane NE, Hochberg MC, Pressman A, et al. Recreational physical activity and the risk of osteoarthritis of the hip in elderly women. *J Rheumatol.* 1999;26:849–854.

31. Croft P, Cooper C, Wickham C, Coggon D. Defining osteoarthritis of the hip for epidemiologic studies. *Am J Epidemiol.* 1990;132: 514–522.

32. Hart DJ, Spector TD. The classification and assessment of osteoarthritis. *Baillieres Clin Rheumatol.* 1995;9:407–432.

33. Saville PD, Dickson J. Age and weight in osteoarthritis of the hip. *Arthritis Rheum.* 1968;11:635–644.

34. Gelber AC, Hochberg MC, Mead LA, et al. Body mass index in young men and the risk of subsequent knee and hip osteoarthritis. *Am J Med.* 1999;107:542–548.

35. Cahuzac JP, Autefage A, Fayolle P, et al. Exaggerated femoral anteversion and acetabular development: experimental study in growing dogs. *J Pediatr Orthop.* 1989;9:163–168.

36. Spyropoulos P, Pisciotta JC, Pavlou KN, et al. Biomechanical gait analysis in obese men. *Arch Phys Med Rehabil.* 1991;72:1065–1070.

37. Hills AP, Parker AW. Gait characteristics of obese children. *Arch Phys Med Rehabil.* 1991;72:403–407.

38. McGraw B, McClenaghan BA, Williams HG, et al. Gait and postural stability in obese and nonobese prepubertal boys. *Arch Phys Med Rehabil.* 2000;81:484–489.

REPRINT

Obesity and Hip Osteoarthritis:
The Weight of the Evidence Is Increasing

Allan C. Gelber, MD

Osteoarthritis affects about 20 million people in the United States (1), with a predilection for particular joint sites in the peripheral skeleton, predominantly the hands, knees, and hips. Osteoarthritis results in substantial morbidity and disability in the elderly, and it is the leading indication for the more than 200,000 knee and hip replacement surgeries performed annually in the United States (2). Notwithstanding the substantial disease burden and the effects on quality of life, there is no curative therapy for osteoarthritis. Conventional treatment reduces symptoms and improves function (3) but does not alter the disease process. Once structural damage to articular cartilage occurs, with joint space narrowing and osteophyte formation, these pathologic changes cannot be reversed by standard therapeutic modalities. Hence, much attention has been invested in improving our understanding of the epidemiology of osteoarthritis and in elucidating which factors predispose to the development of this disorder.

Risk factors for osteoarthritis include those that are fixed (e.g., age, sex, family history, and, possibly, race), as well as those that are amenable, if not in practice, then at least in principle, to modification (e.g., overweight or obesity, physical activity, exercise levels, muscle weakness, and joint injury). To date, the link between overweight or obesity and osteoarthritis has been strongest and most consistently demonstrated for knee osteoarthritis. With regard to the hip joint, epidemiologic data linking obesity with osteoarthritis have been inconsistent. In one population survey from the United States (4), obesity was not associated with unilateral hip osteoarthritis. In contrast, studies from the United Kingdom (5) and Sweden (6,7) reported a positive relation between obesity and hip osteoarthritis. More recently, greater weight and body mass index were associated with a higher incidence of symptomatic hip osteoarthritis in a health plan group (8). Thus, there is increasing evidence suggesting the deleterious role of overweight and obesity in hip osteoarthritis.

Before accepting that increased body weight is a risk factor for hip osteoarthritis, one needs to consider the possible methodologic limitations of the conducted studies. In a recent review (9), relatively few reports were identified from which to infer causality between weight and osteoarthritis. Moreover, only 12 studies, including those cited above, met the eligibility criteria for inclusion in the review. They comprised one cohort study, four case-control studies, and seven cross-sectional studies. However, cross-sectional surveys are limited by ascertainment of exposure and outcome status at the same point in time. Case-control studies may exaggerate the risk of osteoarthritis associated with prior weight because patients with symptomatic hip osteoarthritis may be more likely to overestimate earlier body weight. In contrast, prospective cohort studies determine exposure (obesity) status before the outcome (hip osteoarthritis) develops. It is in this context that the report of Karlson et al. (10), which appears in this issue of the *Journal,* needs to be recognized.

Using data from the Nurses' Health Study, a prospective cohort study of more than 120,000 women, Karlson et al. found that only higher body mass index and older age were associated with an increased risk of osteoarthritis requiring hip replacement surgery (10). In particular, women in the highest category of body mass index had a twofold greater risk of hip arthroplasty, compared with those in the lowest category.

Strengths of their report include the high (>90%) response rate to the biennial questionnaires and the subanalyses to verify the face validity of the outcome. However, the study excluded women with cardiovascular disease, which, given that cardiovascular disease risk factors are highly prevalent among U.S. adults with osteoarthritis (11), may have narrowed the generalizability of the findings. In addition, it is not clear if the weights used to calculate body mass index were obtained at cohort inception (in 1976), or if they were obtained from the 1990 biennial questionnaire (the baseline year for the analyses). If the later values were used, the associated analyses do not allow for a substantial period of time to have elapsed between ascertainment of exposure and development of outcome, as it would had the investigators utilized weight at cohort entry and incident arthroplasty 14 or more years later. In a related fashion, self-reported weight at age 18 years was collected in 1980, when the age range of the cohort was 34 to 59 years. Recalled, rather than actual, weight at age 18 years was used in these analyses; in a separate validity study, these recalled weights correlated strongly with recorded weight in medical records.

A particularly intriguing finding by Karlson et al. was the relation of body mass index at age 18 years to the risk of hip osteoarthritis (10). Moreover, risk estimates at age

Am J Med. 2003;114:158–159.
From the Department of Medicine, Johns Hopkins University School of Medicine, Baltimore, Maryland.

Requests for reprints should be addressed to Allan C. Gelber, MD, Department of Medicine, Johns Hopkins University School of Medicine, 1830 East Monument Street, Suite 7500, Baltimore, Maryland 21205, or agelber@jhmi.edu.

Manuscript submitted August 6, 2002.

0002-9343/03/$–see front matter
doi:10.1016/S0002-9343(02)01548-6

18 years were significantly greater than those for "recent" body mass index, which were reported closer to the date of surgery. This finding complements a previous study that similarly examined the relation of body weight in young adult life to the incidence of hip osteoarthritis among health professionals (12). This other study, however, involved male physicians, and did not find evidence of a link between body weight in the third decade of life and hip osteoarthritis in later life.

It has been estimated that if obesity were eliminated, the prevalence of hip osteoarthritis would decrease by 25% (13). Thus, weight modification could lead to a substantial reduction in the burden of osteoarthritis in weight-bearing joints. The findings by Karlson et al clearly strengthen the argument that greater body weight increases the risk of hip osteoarthritis that is severe enough to warrant replacement surgery, as well as support the position that prevention of osteoarthritis should begin early in life, before the onset of joint pain and before function is compromised.

REFERENCES

1. Lawrence RC, Helmick CG, Arnett FC, et al. Estimates of the prevalence of arthritis and selected musculoskeletal disorders in the United States. *Arthritis Rheum.* 1998;41:778–799.
2. Harris WH, Sledge CB. Total hip and total knee replacement. *N Engl J Med.* 1990;323:725–731.
3. Recommendations for the medical management of osteoarthritis of the hip and knee: 2000 update. American College of Rheumatology Subcommittee on Osteoarthritis Guidelines. *Arthritis Rheum.* 2000;43:1905–1915.
4. Tepper S, Hochberg MC. Factors associated with hip osteoarthritis: data from the First National Health and Nutrition Examination Survey (NHANES-I). *Am J Epidemiol.* 1993;137:1081–1088.
5. Cooper C, Inskip H, Croft P, et al. Individual risk factors for hip osteoarthritis: obesity, hip injury, and physical activity. *Am J Epidemiol.* 1998;147:516–522.
6. Vingard E. Overweight predisposes to coxarthrosis. Body-mass index studied in 239 males with hip arthroplasty. *Acta Orthop Scand.* 1991;62:106–109.
7. Vingard E, Alfredsson L, Malchau H. Lifestyle factors and hip arthrosis. A case referent study of body mass index, smoking and hormone therapy in 503 Swedish women. *Acta Orthop Scand.* 1997;68:216–220.
8. Oliveria SA, Felson DT, Cirillo PA, et al. Body weight, body mass index, and incident symptomatic osteoarthritis of the hand, hip, and knee. *Epidemiology.* 1999;10:161–166.
9. Lievense AM, Bierma-Zeinstra SM, Verhagen AP, et al. Influence of obesity on the development of osteoarthritis of the hip: a systematic review. *Rheumatology (Oxf).* 2002;41:1155–1162.
10. Karlson EW, Mandl LA, Aweh GN, et al. Total hip replacement due to osteoarthritis: the importance of age, obesity, and other modifiable risk factors. *Am J Med.* 2003;114:93–98.
11. Singh G, Miller JD, Lee FH, et al. Prevalence of cardiovascular disease risk factors among US adults with self-reported osteoarthritis: data from the Third National Health and Nutrition Examination Survey. *Am J Manag Care.* 2002;8(suppl):S383–S391.
12. Gelber AC, Hochberg MC, Mead LA, et al. Body mass index in young men and the risk of subsequent knee and hip osteoarthritis. *Am J Med.* 1999;107:542–548.
13. Felson DT, Zhang Y. An update on the epidemiology of knee and hip osteoarthritis with a view to prevention. *Arthritis Rheum.* 1998;41:1343–1355.

NOTES

NOTES

NOTES

NOTES

ISBN 0-929661-88-5
ISSN 1542-135X
Twelfth Printing
Printed in the United States of America

The chart on page 45 is reprinted from American College of Rheumatology Subcommittee on Rheumatoid Arthritis Guidelines. "Guidelines for the Management of Rheumatoid Arthritis." *Arthritis & Rheumatism* Vol. 46, No. 2 (February 2002): 328-346. Copyright © 2002, American College of Rheumatology. Reprinted by permission of Wiley-Liss, Inc., a subsidiary of John Wiley & Sons, Inc.

Karlson, E.W. et al. "Total Hip Replacement Due to Osteoarthritis: The Importance of Age, Obesity, and Other Modifiable Risk Factors." Reprinted with permission from *The American Journal of Medicine* Vol. 114, No. 2 (February 1, 2003): 93-98. Copyright © 2003, Excerpta Medica, Inc.

Gelber, A.C. "Obesity and Hip Osteoarthritis: The Weight of the Evidence Is Increasing." Reprinted with permission from *The American Journal of Medicine* Vol. 114, No. 2 (February 1, 2003): 158-159. Copyright © 2003, Excerpta Medica, Inc.

The Johns Hopkins White Papers are published yearly by Medletter Associates, Inc.

Visit our Web site for information on Johns Hopkins Health After 50 publications, which include White Papers on specific disorders, home medical encyclopedias, consumer reference guides to drugs and medical tests, and our monthly newsletter
The Johns Hopkins Medical Letter: Health After 50.
www.HopkinsAfter50.com

The Johns Hopkins White Papers

Devon Schuyler
Executive Editor

Catherine Richter
Senior Editor

Paul Candon
Senior Writer

Kimberly Flynn
Writer/Researcher

Liz Curry
Editorial Associate

Leslie Maltese-McGill
Copy Editor

Tim Jeffs
Art Director

Vincent Mejia
Graphic Designer

Robert Duckwall
Medical Illustrator

Mary Ellen Bingham
Intern

Johns Hopkins Health After 50 Publications

Rodney Friedman
Editor and Publisher

Thomas Dickey
Editorial Director

Tom Damrauer, M.L.S.
Chief of Information Resources

Helen Mullen
Circulation Director

Tim O'Brien
Circulation Director

Jerry Loo
Product Manager

Darren Leiser
Promotions Coordinator

Joan Mullally
Head of Business Development

The 2004 White Papers

Take Control of Your Medical Condition

Visit us online at www.HopkinsAfter50.com

64B60M

YES, I've placed a check mark next to the White Paper(s) I'd like to receive for $24.95 each. Annual updates on each subject that I have chosen will be offered to me by announcement card. I need do nothing if I want the update to be sent to me automatically. If I do not want it, I will return the announcement card marked "cancel." I may cancel at any time. (Please add $2.95 for domestic, $4.95 for Canadian, and $15.00 for foreign orders to your total to cover shipping and handling.) (Florida residents add sales tax.)

✔ **Please put a check mark next to the White Paper(s) you wish to order.**

001040 ❏ Arthritis	$24.95	008045 ❏ Prostate Disorders	$24.95
003046 ❏ Coronary Heart Disease	$24.95	010041 ❏ Digestive Disorders	$24.95
004044 ❏ Depression and Anxiety	$24.95	011049 ❏ Vision	$24.95
005041 ❏ Diabetes	$24.95	012047 ❏ Back Pain & Osteoporosis	$24.95
006049 ❏ Hypertension and Stroke	$24.95	015040 ❏ Memory	$24.95
007047 ❏ Nutrition and Weight Control for Longevity	$24.95	019042 ❏ Lung Disorders	$24.95
		020040 ❏ Heart Attack Prevention	$24.95

METHOD OF PAYMENT:
(U.S. funds only)

❏ VISA   ❏ Check Enclosed
❏ MasterCard   ❏ Bill Me

Name _____

Address _____

City _____ State ____ Zip ____

Credit Card # _____ Exp. Date ____

Signature _____ Date ____

Money Back Guarantee: If for any reason, you are not satisfied after receipt of your publications, return your purchase within 30 days for a full refund.
Detach and mail this card back to The Johns Hopkins White Papers, P.O. Box 420083, Palm Coast, FL 32142

The 2004 White Papers

Take Control of Your Medical Condition

Visit us online at www.HopkinsAfter50.com

64B60M

YES, I've placed a check mark next to the White Paper(s) I'd like to receive for $24.95 each. Annual updates on each subject that I have chosen will be offered to me by announcement card. I need do nothing if I want the update to be sent to me automatically. If I do not want it, I will return the announcement card marked "cancel." I may cancel at any time. (Please add $2.95 for domestic, $4.95 for Canadian, and $15.00 for foreign orders to your total to cover shipping and handling.) (Florida residents add sales tax.)

✔ **Please put a check mark next to the White Paper(s) you wish to order.**

001040 ❏ Arthritis	$24.95	008045 ❏ Prostate Disorders	$24.95
003046 ❏ Coronary Heart Disease	$24.95	010041 ❏ Digestive Disorders	$24.95
004044 ❏ Depression and Anxiety	$24.95	011049 ❏ Vision	$24.95
005041 ❏ Diabetes	$24.95	012047 ❏ Back Pain & Osteoporosis	$24.95
006049 ❏ Hypertension and Stroke	$24.95	015040 ❏ Memory	$24.95
007047 ❏ Nutrition and Weight Control for Longevity	$24.95	019042 ❏ Lung Disorders	$24.95
		020040 ❏ Heart Attack Prevention	$24.95

METHOD OF PAYMENT:
(U.S. funds only)

❏ VISA   ❏ Check Enclosed
❏ MasterCard   ❏ Bill Me

Name _____

Address _____

City _____ State ____ Zip ____

Credit Card # _____ Exp. Date ____

Signature _____ Date ____

Money Back Guarantee: If for any reason, you are not satisfied after receipt of your publications, return your purchase within 30 days for a full refund.
Detach and mail this card back to The Johns Hopkins White Papers, P.O. Box 420083, Palm Coast, FL 32142

Johns Hopkins White Papers

Fold along this line and tape closed

Johns Hopkins White Papers

Fold along this line and tape closed

2004 WHITE PAPER TITLES

ARTHRITIS 2004 - Covers three common forms of arthritis - osteoarthritis, rheumatoid arthritis, and gout - as well as two other rheumatic diseases: fibromyalgia syndrome and bursitis.

CORONARY HEART DISEASE 2004 - Discusses four problems resulting from coronary heart disease: heart attacks, angina, cardiac arrhythmias, and heart failure.

DEPRESSION and ANXIETY 2004 - Includes major depression, dysthymia, atypical depression, bipolar disorder, seasonal affective disorder, panic disorder, generalized anxiety disorder, obsessive-compulsive disorder, post-traumatic stress disorder, and phobic disorders.

DIABETES 2004 - Shows you how to manage your diabetes and avoid complications such as foot problems and vision changes. Reviews the latest tools for monitoring your blood glucose and the newest medications for controlling it.

DIGESTIVE DISORDERS 2004 - Covers gastroesophageal reflux disease, peptic ulcers, dysphagia, achalasia, Barrett's esophagus, esophageal spasm and stricture, gastritis, gallstones, diarrhea, constipation, Crohn's disease, ulcerative colitis, and colon cancer.

HYPERTENSION and STROKE 2004 - Explains how to treat your high blood pressure and prevent it from harming your health. Also covers the two forms of stroke: ischemic stroke and hemorrhagic stroke.

BACK PAIN and OSTEOPOROSIS 2004 - Addresses back pain due to sprains, strains, and spasms; degenerative changes of the spinal bones and disks; disk herniation; and spinal stenosis. Also covers osteoporosis, a common cause of fractures in the spine and hip.

LUNG DISORDERS 2004 - Includes information on emphysema and chronic bronchitis (together referred to as chronic obstructive pulmonary disease or COPD), asthma, pneumonia, tuberculosis, lung cancer, and sleep apnea.

MEMORY 2004 - Tells you how to keep your memory sharp as you get older, and how to recognize the symptoms of age-associated memory impairment, mild cognitive impairment, and illnesses such as Alzheimer's disease and vascular dementia.

NUTRITION and WEIGHT CONTROL for LONGEVITY 2004 - Gives you the information you need to eat a healthy diet and keep your weight under control. Also explains what to do when the pounds just don't seem to budge.

PROSTATE DISORDERS 2004 - Helps you decide among the various treatment options for prostate cancer, benign prostatic hyperplasia, and prostatitis.

VISION 2004 - Reviews the current knowledge on cataracts, glaucoma, age-related macular degeneration, and diabetic retinopathy. Also discusses ways to cope with low vision.

HEART ATTACK PREVENTION 2004 - Provides up-to-date strategies for preventing a first heart attack, including identifying possible risk factors, the latest screening tests, risk-reducing lifestyle measures, and medications for controlling cholesterol.